Diabetes and Hypoglycemia

How You Can Benefit from Diet, Vitamins, Minerals, Herbs, Exercise, and Other Natural Methods

Michael T. Murray, N.D.

D0974250

PRIMA HEALTH
A Division of Prima Publishing

PRIMA HEALTH and its colophon are trademarks of Prima Communications, Inc.

Library of Congress Cataloging-in-Publication Data

Murray, Michael T.
    Diabetes and Hypoglycemia / Michael T. Murray.
       p.   cm. — (Getting well naturally series)
    Includes bibliographical references and index.
    ISBN 1-55958-426-2 (pbk.) : $9.95
      1. Diabetes—Alternative treatment.   2. Hypoglycemia—Alternative
treatment.   3. Naturopathy.   I. Title.   II. Series.
    RC660.M87   1994
    616.4'6206—dc20
    DNLM/DLC
    for Library of Congress   93–36307
                                         CIP

    99 CC 20 19 18 17 16 15 14
Printed in the United States of America

How to Order:

Single copies may be ordered from Prima Publishing, P.O. Box 1260BK, Rocklin, CA 95677; telephone (916) 632-4400. Quantity discounts are also available. On your letterhead, include information concerning the intended use of the books and the number of books you wish to purchase.

Visit us online at www.primahealth.com

Contents

4 A Closer Look at Hypoglycemia   27

5 Carbohydrates, the Glycemic Index, and Fiber   35

6 Dietary Guidelines and Menu Suggestions   45

Preface

A paradigm is a model used to explain events. As our understanding of the environment and the human body evolves, new paradigms are developed. There is a new paradigm emerging in medicine. The old paradigm viewed the body as a machine; the new paradigm focuses on the interconnectedness of body, mind, emotions, social factors, and the environment in determining the status of health. Rather than relying on drugs and surgery, the new model utilizes natural, noninvasive techniques to promote health and healing.

An interesting aspect of this new paradigm is that it draws from the healing wisdom of many cultures and philosophies, including India (Ayurvedic), China (Taoist), and Greece (Hippocratic). At the forefront of the natural medicine movement is naturopathy, a method of healing that employs various natural means to empower an individual to achieve health. Naturopathic medicine and the emerging paradigm are based largely on four time-tested medical principles. These four principles define the philosophy and foundation of natural medicine whether they are utilized by a naturopath (N.D.), medical doctor

(M.D.), osteopath (D.O.), chiropractor (D.C.), or any other health care provider.

Principle 1. The Healing Power of Nature The human body has considerable power to heal itself. The role of the physician is to facilitate and enhance this process. Increasing evidence supports the contention that the healing process is best enhanced with the aid of natural, nontoxic therapies. Of particular interest is the tremendous healing power of the mind.

Principle 2. First, Do No Harm As Hippocrates said, "Above all else, do no harm." In our current medical system, not only can drugs and surgery be harmful, but so can inappropriate medications and procedures.

Principle 3. Identify and Treat the Cause Of vital importance is the treatment of the underlying causes of a disease rather than suppression of symptoms. Evidence is accumulating that many drug treatments are effective only in suppressing the symptoms, whereas many natural treatments actually address the cause.

Principle 4. The Physician as Teacher The original meaning of the word *doctor* was teacher. The physician's role is to teach the patient about achieving health and avoiding disease.

It is interesting to note that many medical organizations that, in the past, spoke out strongly against naturopathic medicine, now endorse recommendations naturopaths have been making for decades. For example, naturopaths have long extolled the value of eating high-fiber foods; reducing the intake of refined sugars, fats, and food additives; exercising on a regular basis; taking nutritional supplements; and reducing stress.

The acceptance of naturopathy into conventional medicine illustrates the paradigm shift occurring in medicine.

What was once scoffed at is now becoming generally accepted as an effective treatment. In fact, in most instances, the natural alternative offers significant benefit over standard medical practices. It is my wish for the readers of this book that they utilize the recommendations that I have made so that they can live healthier lives.

Acknowledgments

The major blessings in my life are my family and friends. My love for them truly makes life worth living.

Special appreciations to my wife, Gina, for being the answer to so many of my dreams; to my parents, Cliff and Patty Murray, and my grandmother, Pauline Shier, for a strong foundation and a lifetime of good memories; to Bob and Kathy Bunton for their love and acceptance; to Ben Dominitz and everyone at Prima for their commitment and support of my work; to Terry Lemerond and everyone at Enzymatic Therapy for all their friendship and support over the years; to Joseph Pizzorno and the students and faculty at Bastyr College, who have given me encouragement and support; and finally, I am eternally grateful to all the researchers, physicians, and scientists who over the years have strived to better understand the use of natural medicines. Without their work, this series would not exist, and medical progress would halt.

Michael T. Murray, N.D.
July 1993

Before You Read On

- Do not self-diagnose. Proper medical care is critical to good health. If you have symptoms suggestive of an illness, please consult a physician—preferably, a naturopath, holistic physician or osteopath, a chiropractor, or other natural health care specialist.
- If you are currently taking a prescription medication, you absolutely must consult your doctor before discontinuing it.
- If you wish to try the natural approach, discuss it with your physician. Since he or she is most likely unaware of the natural alternatives available, you may need to do some educating. Bring this book along with you to the doctor's office. The natural alternatives being recommended are based upon published studies in medical journals. Key references are provided if your physician wants additional information.
- Remember, although many natural alternatives, such as nutritional supplements and plant-based medicines, are effective on their own, they work even better if they are part of a comprehensive natural treatment plan that focuses on diet and lifestyle.

1

Introduction to Diabetes and Hypoglycemia

A lack as well as an excess of blood sugar (glucose) can be devastating. For this reason, the body strives to maintain blood sugar levels within a narrow range through the coordinated effort of several glands and their hormones. If these control mechanisms are disrupted, diabetes (high blood sugar) or hypoglycemia (low blood sugar) may result.

Ideally, the body responds to the rise in blood glucose after meals by secreting insulin, a hormone produced by the beta cells of the pancreas. Insulin lowers blood glucose by increasing the rate at which cells throughout the body absorb glucose. Declines in blood glucose—which occur during food deprivation or exercise—cause the release of glucagon, a hormone produced by the alpha cells of the pancreas. Glucagon stimulates the release of glucose stored as glycogen in body tissues (especially the liver). If the blood sugar level falls sharply or if a person is angry or frightened, the result may be the release of epinephrine (adrenaline) and corticosteroids (one of the most important being cortisol) by the adrenal glands. These hormones quickly break down stored glucose to provide the extra energy the body needs during a crisis or some other time of increased need.

Unfortunately, the response of the body is not always ideal. For example, the diet and lifestyle of many people— Americans in particular—stress the natural glucose-control mechanisms. As a result, diabetes and hypoglycemia are among the most common of American diseases.

What Is Diabetes?

Diabetes is a chronic disorder of carbohydrate, fat, and protein metabolism, characterized by elevation of the blood sugar level after fasting. Diabetes greatly increases the risk of loss of nerve function as well as the risk of heart disease, stroke, and kidney disease. Diabetes can occur when the pancreas does not secrete enough insulin or if the cells of the body become resistant to insulin. Insulin is a hormone that promotes the uptake of blood sugar by the cells of the body. When there is not enough insulin or when cells lack sensitivity to it, blood sugar cannot get into the cells. This can lead to serious complications.

The classic symptoms of diabetes are frequent urination, excessive thirst and appetite. Because these symptoms are not too terribly serious, many people with diabetes do not seek medical care. In fact, of the more than 10 million Americans with diabetes, fewer than half know they have diabetes or ever consult a physician.

Diabetes is divided into two major categories: type I and type II. Type I, or insulin-dependent diabetes mellitus (IDDM), occurs most often in children and adolescents. It is associated with complete destruction of the beta cells of the pancreas, which manufacture insulin. Those with type I diabetes must receive doses of insulin throughout their lives to control their blood sugar level. The type I diabetic must learn how to manage his or her blood sugar on a day-by-day basis, modifying insulin types and dosage schedules as necessary, according to the results of regular blood sugar testing. About 10% of all diabetics are type I. What ultimately destroys the beta cells of the pancreas are antibodies produced by white blood cells. Antibodies are designed to seek out and destroy infecting organisms, such as viruses and bacteria. However, in some diseases, antibodies develop that target the body's own tissues. These diseases are referred to as autoimmune diseases. Type I diabetes appears to have an autoimmune component at its origin, because antibodies for beta cells are present in 75% of all cases. In the "normal" population, these antibodies are present in only 0.5% to 2.0% of cases. It is probable that antibodies for beta cells develop in response to cell destruction caused by other mechanisms (chemicals, free radicals, viruses, food allergies, and so on). It appears that normal individuals either do not develop as severe an antibody reaction as do those who become diabetics or that normal people are better able to repair the damage caused by antibodies once it occurs.

The onset of type II, or non–insulin dependent diabetes mellitus (NIDDM), usually occurs after the person who develops it is 40 years of age. Up to 90% of all diabetics are type II diabetics. Typically, the insulin level of these people is elevated, indicating that body cells have lost sensitivity to insulin. Obesity is a major contributing factor to this loss of sensitivity. Approximately 90% of individuals with type II diabetes are obese. For most of these people, achieving ideal body weight is associated with restoration of normal blood sugar levels.

In type II diabetes, diet is of primary importance. Dietary treatment must be tried diligently before a drug is used. Most type II diabetes can be controlled by diet alone. Despite a high success rate with dietary intervention, however, many eager physicians use drugs or insulin instead.

Table 1.1 cites the differences between type I and type II diabetes.

Other types of diabetes include secondary diabetes (a form that is secondary to certain conditions and syndromes, such as pancreatic disease, hormone disturbances, drugs, and malnutrition), gestational diabetes (glucose intolerance occurring during pregnancy), and impaired glucose tolerance (a condition that includes pre-diabetic, chemical, latent, borderline, subclinical, and asymptomatic diabetes). Individuals with impaired glucose tolerance have a blood glucose level and glucose tolerance test results that are intermediate, between normal test results and those that are clearly abnormal. (You will learn about the glucose tolerance test in Chapter 2.) In addition, many practitioners consider reactive hypoglycemia a pre-diabetic condition.

Table 1.1   Differences Between Type I and Type II Diabetes

Features	Type I	Type II
Age at onset	Usually under 40	Usually over 40
Proportion of all diabetics	Less than 10%	Up to 90%
Seasonal trend	Fall and winter	None
Family history	Uncommon	Common
Appearance of symptoms	Rapid	Slow
Obesity at onset	Uncommon	Common
Insulin level	Decreased	Variable
Insulin resistance	Occasional	Often
Treatment with insulin	Always	Usually not required
Beta cells	Decreased	Variable
Abnormally high levels of ketones and lactic acid in blood (ketoacidosis)*	Frequent	Rare
Complications	Frequent	Frequent

*A ketone is a weak acid produced by the breakdown of fat by-products.

What Is Hypoglycemia?

Hypoglycemia results from the faulty metabolism of carbohydrates (sugars). The body strives to maintain a blood sugar level within a narrow range, primarily to ensure the brain a constant supply of glucose. Because glucose is the primary fuel for the brain, when the level of glucose is too low, the brain is affected first. Symptoms of hypoglycemia can range from mild to severe and include headache; depression, anxiety, irritability, and other psychological disturbances; blurred vision; excessive sweating; confusion; incoherent speech; bizarre behavior; and convulsions.

Hypoglycemia is divided into two main categories: reactive hypoglycemia and fasting hypoglycemia. Reactive hypoglycemia is the most common type. It is characterized by the development of symptoms of hypoglycemia from 2 to 4 hours after a meal. Reactive hypoglycemia may also result from the use of certain drugs.

Fasting hypoglycemia is extremely rare. It usually only appears in severe disease states, such as those involving pancreatic tumors, extensive liver damage, prolonged starvation, and various cancers.

The Diabetes-Hypoglycemia Link

Blood sugar problems are strongly associated with the so-called Western diet. This diet is rich in refined sugar, fat, and animal products and low in dietary fiber. It is widely accepted that refined carbohydrates are the most important contributing factor to diabetes and reactive hypoglycemia (as well as obesity). Refined sugars are quickly absorbed into the bloodstream, causing a rapid rise in blood sugar. The body's response to this is to greatly increase the secretion of insulin by the pancreas. The excessive secretion of insulin drives the blood sugar level down and often causes the symptoms of hypoglycemia.

In response to the rapid fall in blood sugar, the adrenal glands secrete epinephrine (adrenaline), which causes a rapid increase in the blood sugar level. In time, the adrenal glands become "exhausted" by the repeated stress and cannot mount an appropriate response. This lack of response leads to reactive hypoglycemia. If blood sugar control mechanisms are further stressed, the body will eventually become insensitive to insulin or the pancreas will also become exhausted and the reactive hypoglycemia will turn into diabetes.

Obviously, the most critical component of diabetes and hypoglycemia treatment or prevention is the avoidance of refined sugar. However, by utilizing the natural approach that the following chapters will discuss, much more can be done.

Chapter Summary

The body strives to maintain a blood sugar level that is within a normal range. When blood sugar control mechanisms are disturbed, either diabetes or hypoglycemia may occur. Blood sugar disorders are quite common in American society because of Americans' excessive consumption of sugar and fat and the low intake of dietary fiber.

2

Diagnosis of Diabetes
and Hypoglycemia '

I f you suspect that you have a problem with blood sugar control, it is vital that you see a physician for proper diagnosis. The standard methods of diagnosing diabetes and hypoglycemia involve the measurement of blood glucose levels. After a fast the normal blood glucose level is between 70 and 105 milligrams per deciliter (mg/dL). In general, if on two separate occasions a person has a fasting blood glucose measurement greater than 140 milligrams per deciliter, the diagnosis is diabetes; if the level is below 50 milligrams per deciliter, the diagnosis is fasting hypoglycemia.[1]

The Oral Glucose Tolerance Test

The oral glucose tolerance test (GTT) is used in the diagnosis of both diabetes and reactive hypoglycemia, although it is rarely required for diabetes. After the subject fasts for at least 12 hours, a baseline blood glucose measurement is made. Then the subject drinks a very sweet liquid containing

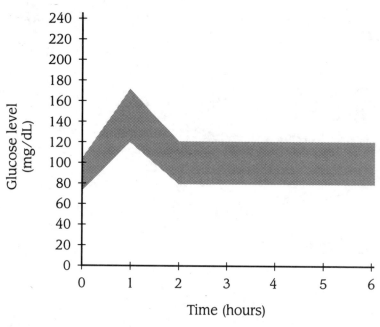

Figure 2.1   The normal range for the oral GTT

glucose. The blood sugar level is rechecked at 30 minutes, 1 hour, and then hourly for up to 6 hours. Basically, if the blood sugar level rises to more than 200 milligrams per deciliter, the test indicates diabetes. If the level falls below 50 milligrams per deciliter, the test indicates reactive hypoglycemia. Figure 2.1 shows oral GTT results in the normal range. Figure 2.2 provides additional information about interpreting GTT results.

The Glucose-Insulin Tolerance Test

Measuring blood sugar levels alone is often not enough to diagnose blood sugar disorders. This is especially true in hypoglycemia, because symptoms of hypoglycemia can occur in individuals having blood glucose levels well above 50 milligrams per deciliter.[2] Many of the symptoms linked

Normal: No elevation greater than 160 mg; below 150 mg at the end of 1st hour, below 120 mg at the end of 2nd hour

Flat: No variation more or less than 20 mg from fasting value

Pre-diabetic: Over 120 mg at the end of 2nd hour

Diabetic: Over 180 mg during the 1st hour, 200 mg or higher at the end of 1st hour, and 150 mg or higher at the end of 2nd hour

Reactive hypoglycemia: A normal response curve for 2–3 hours, followed by a decrease of 20 mg or more from the fasting level during the final hours

Probable reactive hypoglycemia: A normal response curve for 2–3 hours, followed by a decrease of 10–20 mg from the fasting level during the final hours

Flat hypoglycemia: An elevation of 20 mg or less, followed by a decrease of at least 20 mg below fasting level

Pre-diabetic hypoglycemia: A 2-hour response identical to the pre-diabetic, but a hypoglycemic response during the final 3 hours

Hyperinsulinism: A marked hypoglycemic response, with a value of less than 50 mg during the 3rd, 4th, or 5th hour

Figure 2.2   GTT response criteria

to hypoglycemia appear to be a result of increases in insulin or epinephrine. Therefore, it has been recommended that insulin or epinephrine be measured at the same time, since symptoms often correlate better with elevations of these hormones than with glucose levels.[3,4] Several studies have shown that the glucose-insulin tolerance test (G-ITT) leads to a greater sensitivity in the diagnosis of both hypoglycemia and diabetes than the standard GTT.[4,5]

The G-ITT is a standard 6-hour GTT coupled with the measurement of insulin levels. The G-ITT appears to be one of the best diagnostic indicators for faulty sugar metabolism.[5] As many as two-thirds of subjects with suspected diabetes or hypoglycemia, subjects who have normal GTTs, demonstrate abnormal G-ITTs. The downside to the G-ITT is that it tends to be very costly. A G-ITT costs around $200; a standard GTT usually costs less than $30. Despite the high

---

Pattern 1: Normal fasting insulin is 0–30 units. Peak insulin at 30–60 min. The combined insulin values for the 2nd and 3rd hours is less than 60 units. This pattern is considered normal.

Pattern 2: Normal fasting insulin. Peak at 30–60 min, with a delayed return to normal. Second- and third-hour levels between 60 and 100 units are usually associated with hypoglycemia and considered border-line for diabetes. Values greater than 100 units definitely indicate diabetes.

Pattern 3: Normal fasting insulin. Peak in 2nd or 3rd hour instead of 30–60 min. Definite indication of diabetes.

Pattern 4: High insulin after fasting. Definite indication of diabetes.

Pattern 5: Low insulin response. All tested values for insulin are less than 30. If this response is associated with elevated blood sugar levels, the result is probable insulin-dependent diabetes (juvenile pattern).

Figure 2.3   G-ITT response criteria

price, the G-ITT and other diagnostic tests are often appropriate. Figure 2.3 provides additional information about interpreting G-ITT results.

The Hypoglycemic Index

Another laboratory parameter that can aid in the diagnosis of hypoglycemia, especially the borderline case, is the so-called hypoglycemic index. This value is determined by dividing the decrease in the blood glucose level (during the 90-minute period before it reaches the lowest point) by the value of the lowest point. A hypoglycemic index greater than 0.8 usually indicates reactive hypoglycemia.

The Hypoglycemia Questionnaire

When all is considered (especially cost), in many cases the most useful tool in the diagnosis of hypoglycemia remains

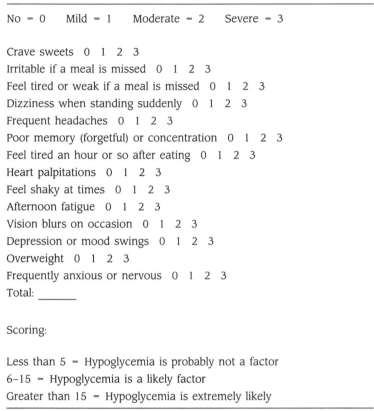

No = 0   Mild = 1   Moderate = 2   Severe = 3

Crave sweets 0 1 2 3
Irritable if a meal is missed 0 1 2 3
Feel tired or weak if a meal is missed 0 1 2 3
Dizziness when standing suddenly 0 1 2 3
Frequent headaches 0 1 2 3
Poor memory (forgetful) or concentration 0 1 2 3
Feel tired an hour or so after eating 0 1 2 3
Heart palpitations 0 1 2 3
Feel shaky at times 0 1 2 3
Afternoon fatigue 0 1 2 3
Vision blurs on occasion 0 1 2 3
Depression or mood swings 0 1 2 3
Overweight 0 1 2 3
Frequently anxious or nervous 0 1 2 3
Total: _____

Scoring:

Less than 5 = Hypoglycemia is probably not a factor
6–15 = Hypoglycemia is a likely factor
Greater than 15 = Hypoglycemia is extremely likely

Figure 2.4   The hypoglycemia questionnaire

the hypoglycemia questionnaire, which assesses symptoms. Figure 2.4 presents the hypoglycemia questionnaire.

Glycosylated Hemoglobin

Proteins that have glucose molecules attached to them are said to be glycosylated. The diabetic has a level of glycosylated proteins that is several times higher than normal. The measurement of the level of glycosylated hemoglobin

(hemoglobin A_{1c}) is used for monitoring blood sugar levels over a long period. Normally, 5% to 7% of hemoglobin is combined with glucose. Mild elevations in blood sugar result in a glycosylated hemoglobin A_{1c} concentration of 8% to 10%; severe elevations may result in concentrations of up to 20%.

The average life span of a red blood cell is 120 days. A completed assay of glycosylated hemoglobin results in time-averaged values for blood glucose over the preceding 2 to 4 months, thus providing a simple, useful method for assessing treatment effectiveness and patient compliance. Glycosylated hemoglobin can also be used in some cases to diagnose diabetes. Although the oral GTT is more sensitive than an assay of glycosylated hemoglobin, it is also more stressful to the patient. Because an elevated glycosylated hemoglobin level almost always indicates diabetes, many physicians simply measure the level of glycosylated hemoglobin rather than subject patients, particularly pregnant women, to the stress of a GTT.

Chapter Summary

A diagnosis of diabetes or hypoglycemia is often based on measurements of blood glucose levels after fasting or during a GTT. Measuring the insulin level along with the glucose level during a GTT greatly increases diagnostic sensitivity. In the case of hypoglycemia, the best diagnostic aid may be the hypoglycemia questionnaire. If diabetes is suspected and the stress of a GTT is to be avoided, measuring the level of glycosylated hemoglobin may provide an adequate diagnosis.

3

A Closer Look at Diabetes

Diabetes is a very serious disorder that needs to be treated effectively. Current medical treatment has undoubtedly helped many diabetics to live healthier and longer than they would have without treatment. However, there is room for substantial improvement in the medical approach. Although the diagnosis of diabetes is no longer an immediate death sentence, it still carries with it a restricted daily life and an increased risk of premature death and disability. This chapter will examine the current medical treatment of diabetes to control the blood sugar level and prevent the complications of diabetes.

Current Medical Treatment of Type I Diabetes

There is no question that a type I diabetic requires insulin. Insulin preparations have been used in the treatment of diabetes since 1922. Since insulin is not absorbed orally, it must be injected. Insulin preparations come in concentrations of 100 units per milliliter (U/100) and 500 units per milliliter (U/500). Preparations differ in their source (cows, pigs, or synthetic chemicals designed to resemble human insulin), duration of action (rapid, intermediate, and long-acting), and solubility (crystalline versus soluble). Synthetic insulin is gaining wider acceptance as the preferred substance.

Conventional insulin therapy involves administering crystalline insulin, usually a mixture of rapid- and inter-mediate-acting insulin, once or twice daily. This method is being replaced by intensified insulin therapy in which the insulin is given in increasingly sophisticated and complex regimens. The reason? Evidence demonstrates that intensified insulin therapy significantly reduces the development of the chronic complications of diabetes (discussed later in this chapter).[1] Intensified insulin therapy is designed to mimic, as closely as possible, the continuous variations in plasma insulin levels produced by a healthy pancreas.

The methods of applying intensified insulin therapy are multiple daily injections (3 to 5 injections per day) or the use of the "insulin pump" to administer a continuous supply of insulin. Use of the insulin pump involves a syringe, which is filled with soluble insulin. The syringe, which looks like a ballpoint pen, is connected via a hollow flexible hose to a syringe. The needle of the syringe is inserted into a site on the abdomen. The pump part of the mechanism slowly presses the plunger of the syringe so that it delivers a constant trickle of soluble insulin. Fifteen minutes prior to a meal, the diabetic can press the pump manually to release a burst of insulin.

The insulin pump approximates the natural levels of insulin and is the best of currently available techniques, but it is not without drawbacks. The device must be worn constantly and can be an irritation. The patient must be highly motivated to monitor blood sugar levels quite closely. The pump method involves a greater risk for hypoglycemia than the method of multiple daily injections, and not all physicians are familiar enough with the pump method to advise patients in its use. Regardless of the type of insulin therapy used, the treatment of diabetes must include proper diet and lifestyle.

Current Medical Treatment of Type II Diabetes

When type II diabetes cannot be controlled satisfactorily with diet therapy, many medical doctors use drugs known as oral hypoglycemic agents. These agents are sulfa drugs called sulfonylureas. They appear to stimulate the secretion of insulin by the pancreas as well as enhance the sensitivity of body tissues to insulin. Some common examples of this class of drugs include:

Chlorpropamide (Diabinese)

Glipizide (Glucotrol)

Glyburide (DiaBeta, Micronase)

Tolazamide (Tolinase)

Tolbutamide (Orinase)

As a group, these drugs are not very effective. After three months of continual treatment at an adequate dosage, sulfonylureas fail to adequately control blood sugar in about 40% of cases. Furthermore, these drugs generally lose their effectiveness over time. After an initial period of success, these drugs will fail to produce a positive effect in about 30% of cases. The overall success rate of adequate control by long-term use of sulfonylureas is no more than 30% at best.

In addition to being of limited value, there is evidence to indicate that these drugs actually produce harmful long-term side effects. For example, a famous study conducted by the University Group Diabetes Program on the long-term effects of tolbutamide showed that the rate of death due to heart attack or stroke was 2½ times greater for the group that used sulfonylureas than that for the group that controlled type II diabetes by diet alone.[2]

The major side effect of sulfonylureas is hypoglycemia. Other possible side effects include allergic skin reactions, headache, fatigue, indigestion, nausea and vomiting, and liver damage. Because of the high risk of side effects, sulfonylureas have to be used with extreme caution. They should not be used in situations involving:

Pregnancy

Known allergy to sulfa drugs

Infection, injury, or surgery

Long-term corticosteroid use

What is more, sulfonylureas must be used with extreme caution in the treatment of the very old, alcoholics, those taking multiple drugs, and those with impaired liver or kidney function.

In some cases, physicians prescribe insulin in addition to sulfonylureas. Since most type II diabetics are obese and secrete large amounts of insulin each day (to overcome the resistance that body cells have developed to insulin), additional insulin usually provides little help. To give you an idea just how much insulin an obese type II diabetic secretes, just look at these numbers: Healthy individuals secrete approximately 31 units of insulin daily; the obese type II diabetic secretes an average of 114 units daily. This amount is nearly four times normal. In contrast to obese type II individuals, lean type II individuals produce about 14 units daily; individuals with type I diabetes secrete only 4 units of insulin daily. If a diabetic is overproducing insulin, it makes more sense to work on increasing the *sensitivity* to insulin by following the recommendations given throughout this book.

Prevention of the Complications of Diabetes

Diabetes gives rise to numerous complications. The likelihood of developing complications, whether acute or chronic, is ultimately a reflection of the level of blood sugar control. A large body of evidence indicates that the better the blood sugar control, the less likely the development of complications. Therefore, monitoring and controlling blood sugar is critical to the prevention of the major diabetic complications. The advent of home glucose monitoring has brought about major improvement in the care of diabetes. Typically, the diabetic obtains a blood sample by using a simple spring-triggered device equipped with a disposable lancet. The best sites to take samples are the sides of outside fingers and toes. (The diabetic must take care to avoid the nail beds.) The patient determines the glucose level by placing the sample on a reagent strip and then placing the strip into a small machine known as a glucometer. The glucometer displays the glucose level. There are also reagent strips that give satisfactory results by visual inspection. The patient compares the strip to a colored scale to learn the level of blood sugar.

Another valuable tool in blood sugar control is the assay for glycosylated hemoglobin. (Chapter 2 described this assay.) Normally, 5% to 7% of hemoglobin A found in red blood cells is combined with glucose. Mild hyperglycemia results when the concentration of glycosylated hemoglobin is 8% to 10%. Severe hyperglycemia may result in concentrations up to 20%. Since the average life span of a red blood cell is 120 days, this assay is believed to represent time-averaged values for blood glucose over the 2 to 4 months before the test. An assay of glycosylated hemoglobin is a simple, useful method for assessing blood sugar control over a relatively long period.

In addition to controlling and monitoring blood sugar levels, dietary practices, essential nutrients, medicinal plants, and lifestyle factors are critical in preventing diabetic complications. These topics are discussed in the chapters to follow.

Acute Complications

Diabetics are susceptible to three major acute complications: hypoglycemia, diabetic ketoacidosis (which primarily affects type I diabetics), and nonketogenic hyperosmolar syndrome (which primarily affects type II diabetics).

Hypoglycemia   The problem of hypoglycemia is much more common in type I versus type II diabetes because the type I diabetic is injecting insulin. Taking too much insulin, missing a meal, or overexercising can result in hypoglycemia. It is imperative that the patient and his or her physician work together so that insulin dosages can be gauged correctly.

Daytime hypoglycemic episodes are usually accompanied by the following symptoms: sweating, nervousness, tremor, and hunger. Nighttime hypoglycemia may be without symptoms or manifest as night sweats, unpleasant dreams, or early-morning headache.

In response to hypoglycemia, there is an increase in circulating levels of hormones—such as epinephrine, norepinephrine, growth hormone, and cortisol—that raise blood glucose levels. As a result, blood glucose often rebounds and leads to hyperglycemia. This phenomenon is commonly referred to as the Somogyi phenomenon. It is very important to recognize this response when monitoring insulin needs. The Somogyi phenomenon should be suspected whenever there are wide swings in blood glucose over short periods of time during the day. For example, a blood glucose level of 70 milligrams per deciliter before breakfast and 400 milligrams per deciliter before lunch suggest early-morning hypoglycemia with postbreakfast hyperglycemia due to increased counter-regulatory hormone activity. The advent of the improved insulin therapy, the insulin pump, and home glucose monitors have led to better blood glucose control and a decreased frequency of the Somogyi phenomenon.

Diabetic Ketoacidosis   Another acute complication more likely to occur in the type I diabetic is ketoacidosis—a condition caused by a lack of insulin, which leads to a buildup of ketones, or ketoacids (an acid produced by the breakdown of fat by-products). If progressive, ketoacidosis can result in numerous metabolic problems and cause a coma. The coma is usually preceded by a day or more of increased urination and thirst as well as marked fatigue, nausea, and vomiting. Since ketoacidosis is potentially a medical emergency, its prompt recognition is imperative. Diabetics can use a simple urine dipstick at home to measure the level of ketones in the urine.

Nonketogenic Hyperosmolar Syndrome   With a mortality rate of over 50%, nonketogenic hyperosmolar syndrome constitutes a true medical emergency. It is usually the result of profound dehydration secondary to deficient fluid intake or precipitating events such as pneumonia; burns; stroke; a recent operation; or certain drugs, such as phenytoin, diazoxide, glucocorticoids, or diuretics.

The onset of the syndrome may be insidious over a period of days or weeks, with symptoms of weakness, increased urination and thirst, and progressively worse signs of dehydration (weight loss, loss of skin elasticity, dry mucous membranes, rapid heartbeat, and low blood pressure).

The Causes of Chronic Complications of Diabetes

The two primary causes of most chronic complications of diabetes are glycosylated proteins and the accumulation of sorbitol.

Glycosylated Proteins   The binding of glucose to proteins, a process referred to as glycosylation, leads to changes in the structure and function of many body proteins. For example, glycosylated molecules of low-density lipoprotein (LDL), which are found in high levels in diabetics, do not bind to LDL receptors or shut off cholesterol synthesis. In diabetes, excessive glycosylation also occurs with albumin (a blood protein) and the proteins of the red blood cell, lens, and myelin sheath. This glycosylation causes abnormal structures and functions of involved cells and tissues and contributes greatly to the complications of diabetes.

Sorbitol   Sorbitol is a by-product of glucose metabolism. It is formed within the cell with the help of an enzyme, aldose reductase. In nondiabetic individuals, sorbitol can be metabolized, with the help of another enzyme (polyol dehydrogenase), into fructose. This conversion to fructose allows the sorbitol to be excreted from the cell if concentrations increase. Unfortunately, in the diabetic with routine hyperglycemia, sorbitol accumulates and plays a major role in the development of chronic complications of diabetes.

The mechanism by which sorbitol is involved in the development of diabetic complications is best understood by considering its involvement in cataract formation. Although the lens does not have any blood vessels, it is an actively metabolizing tissue that continuously repairs itself. Since the lens membranes are virtually impermeable to sorbitol and lack the enzyme polyol dehydrogenase, sorbitol accumulates to high concentrations. These high concentrations persist even if the glucose level returns to normal. The accumulation of sorbitol creates an osmotic gradient—water is drawn into the cells to maintain an equal concentration of water inside and outside the cells. As the water is pulled in, the cell must release small molecules—such as amino acids, inositol, glutathione, niacin, vitamin C, magnesium, and potassium—to maintain osmotic balance. Since these molecules protect the lens from damage, their loss results in an increased susceptibility to lens damage. As a result, the delicate protein fibers within the lens become opaque and a cataract forms.

Chronic Complications of Diabetes

On a long-term basis, several major complications may affect the health of the diabetic. These include atherosclerosis, diabetic retinopathy, diabetic neuropathy, diabetic nephropathy, and diabetic foot ulcers.

Atherosclerosis   Atherosclerosis is the buildup of plaque in the walls of arteries. The condition leads to heart attack, stroke, and other circulatory disturbances. Atherosclerosis is by far the major cause of death in the United States. All together, heart disease, stroke, and other diseases caused by atherosclerosis are responsible for at least 43% of all U.S. deaths. The diabetic faces a risk of dying prematurely of atherosclerosis that is 2 or 3 times higher than that of the nondiabetic.

Because of the increased risk of death due to atherosclerosis, the diabetic must be aggressive in reducing the risk factors linked to heart attack and stroke. Foremost is the reduction of blood cholesterol. The evidence overwhelmingly demonstrates that an elevated cholesterol level greatly increases the risk of death due to heart disease. The first step in reducing the risk of heart disease is to keep total blood cholesterol below 200 milligrams per deciliter.

Not all cholesterol is bad; it serves many vital functions in the body, including the manufacture of sex hormones and bile acids. Without cholesterol, many body processes would not function properly. Cholesterol is transported in the blood by molecules known as lipoproteins. Cholesterol bound to low-density lipoprotein, or LDL, is often referred to as bad cholesterol; cholesterol bound to high-density lipoprotein, or HDL, is referred to as good cholesterol. LDL cholesterol increases the risk of heart disease, stroke, and high blood pressure. HDL cholesterol actually protects against heart disease.

LDL transports cholesterol to the tissues. HDL, on the other hand, transports cholesterol to the liver for metabolism and excretion from the body. Therefore the HDL-to-LDL ratio largely determines whether cholesterol is being deposited into tissues or broken down and excreted. The risk of heart disease can be reduced dramatically by lowering LDL cholesterol while raising HDL cholesterol. Research has shown that, for every 1% drop in the LDL cholesterol level, the risk of heart attack drops by 2%. Conversely, for every 1% increase in the HDL level, the risk of heart attack drops 3% to 4%.

In addition to keeping an eye on the cholesterol level, the diabetic must also keep the level of triglycerides (blood fats, or lipids, that increase the risk of heart disease) in the proper range. Both cholesterol and triglycerides are usually elevated in diabetes. Table 3.1 presents recommended levels of these substances.

The most important approach to lowering LDL cholesterol is to follow a healthy diet and lifestyle. The dietary changes are simple: Eat less saturated fat and cholesterol by reducing or eliminating the amount of animal products in the diet; increase the consumption of fiber-rich plant foods (fruits, vegetables, grains, and legumes); and lose

Table 3.1   Recommended Blood Cholesterol and Triglyceride Levels

Total cholesterol	Less than 200 mg/dL
LDL cholesterol	Less than 130 mg/dL
HDL cholesterol	Greater than 35 mg/dL
Triglycerides	50–150 mg/dL

Table 3.2   Food Choices for Lowering Cholesterol

Eat Fewer	Substitute
Red meats	Fish and white meat of poultry
Hamburgers and hot dogs	Soy-based alternatives
Eggs	Tofu, egg substitutes
High-fat dairy products	Lowfat or nonfat dairy products
Butter, lard, and other saturated fats	Vegetable oils
Ice cream, pies, cake, cookies, etc.	Fruits
Refined cereals, white bread, etc.	Whole grains, whole-wheat bread
Fried foods, fatty snack foods	Vegetables, fresh salads
High-sodium salt, salty foods	High-potassium salt, low-sodium foods
Coffee and soft drinks	Herbal teas, fresh fruit and vegetable juices

weight, if necessary. The lifestyle changes include getting regular aerobic exercise, stopping smoking, and reducing or eliminating the consumption of coffee (both caffeinated and decaffeinated).

The importance of even simple alterations in diet can be quite significant. In one study participants ate two medium-sized carrots daily at breakfast. After three weeks, the participants' LDL cholesterol level had been reduced by 11%.[3] Table 3.2 details some simple food choices that can lead to dramatic changes in your cholesterol level and level of health.

Chapter 10 will present in-depth recommendations for preventing and reversing (yes, *reversing*) atherosclerosis.

Diabetic Neuropathy   Among the most frequent complications of long-term diabetes, diabetic neuropathy (nerve disorder) can result in loss of nerve function, tingling sensations, numbness, pain, and muscle weakness. Occasionally neuropathy can affect "deep" nerves and result in decreased heart function, alternating bouts of diarrhea and constipation, inability to empty the bladder, and impotence. The earliest and best-measured signs of diabetic neuropathy are decreased sensory and nerve conduction velocities. Substantial evidence suggests that diabetic neuropathy is due, in part, to sorbitol accumulation. In rats, increasing the sorbitol concentration in the sciatic nerve is directly related to decreasing nerve conduction velocity, possibly as a result of a decreased concentration of *myo*-inositol (a vitamin of the B complex).[4] Sorbitol accumulation leads to *myo*-inositol loss. Although some studies have shown that inositol supplementation improves nerve conduction velocity, addressing the underlying accumulation of sorbitol is of greater importance.[5]

Diabetic Retinopathy   A serious eye disease that can result in blindness, diabetic retinopathy is still the leading cause of blindness in the United States. Of type I diabetics, 1 in 20 develops retinopathy; 1 in 15 type II diabetics develops it. The continued development of laser therapy will undoubtedly reduce the number of people that go blind as a result of diabetes, but laser therapy should be limited to severe cases. The occasional side effects of laser therapy (vitreous hemorrhage, vitreous contraction with retinal detachment, macular edema, and visual field loss) may outweigh its benefits for patients with mild forms of retinopathy.

Diabetic Nephropathy   Kidney disease related to diabetes is called diabetic nephropathy. It is a common complication and a leading cause of death among diabetics. Periodic monitoring of the levels of blood urea nitrogen (BUN), uric acid, and creatinine and of creatinine clearance is vitally important in determining kidney function.

Diabetic Foot Ulcers Atherosclerosis and loss of nerve function can decrease the supply of blood and oxygen to the feet. Lack of blood and oxygen is the key factor in the development of diabetic foot ulcers. Foot ulcers are largely preventable through proper foot care, the avoidance of injury, abstinence from tobacco in any form, and employing methods to improve circulation in the feet. Proper foot care includes keeping the feet clean, dry, and warm and wearing only well-fitting shoes. Avoiding tobacco is important, because tobacco constricts blood vessels and can lead to serious disease in diabetics. Circulation can be improved by not sitting with the legs crossed or in other positions that compromise blood flow and by massaging the feet and ankles with light pressure in an upward direction.

Chapter Summary

Diabetes is a serious disease that requires proper treatment. In type I diabetes, insulin is required. Intensified insulin therapy is becoming the preferred method of treating type I diabetes because it resembles the natural secretion of insulin. The current medical treatment of type II diabetes involves diet and oral hypoglycemic agents. Unfortunately, oral hypoglycemic agents are not very effective and may have many side effects. The goal of medical treatment is to keep blood sugar levels within the normal range and to prevent the complications of diabetes.

4

A Closer Look at Hypoglycemia

I n the 1970s, hypoglycemia was a popular diagnosis for a long list of symptoms. Basically, every symptom on the hypoglycemia questionnaire (Figure 2.4) was linked to hypoglycemia. Although all these symptoms *may* be due to hypoglycemia, there are obviously other causes of them. Since hypoglycemia is not talked about as much nowadays as in the '70s, the question is: Has hypoglycemia been replaced by more exciting labels or have we simply forgot about it as a cause of these symptoms? I think the answer is a combination of both.

During the 1970s there were a number of popular books about hypoglycemia. *Sugar Blues* by William Dufty, *Hope for Hypoglycemia* by Broda Barnes, and *Sweet and Dangerous* by John Yudkin were among the most popular. These books generated tremendous public interest in hypoglycemia and sugar intake; and they were met by much skepticism in the medical community. Editorials in the *Journal of the American Medical Association* and the *New England*

Journal of Medicine denounced this public interest and tried to invalidate the existence of hypoglycemia.[1,2]

In the 1990s, there is an ever-increasing amount of new information about the role that refined carbohydrates and faulty blood sugar control play in many disease processes. Many new words or descriptions are now used to describe the complex hormonal fluxes that are largely a result of the ingestion of too much refined carbohydrate. For example, the term *syndrome X* has recently been introduced to describe a cluster of abnormalities that largely owe their existence to a high intake of refined carbohydrate. These abnormalities can lead to hypoglycemia, excessive insulin secretion, and glucose intolerance. These, in turn, can cause diminished insulin sensitivity and, eventually, high blood pressure, elevated cholesterol, and obesity. Ultimately, syndrome X abnormalities can lead to type II diabetes.[3] Syndrome X will be discussed in more detail in Chapter 10, "Syndrome X and Cardiovascular Disease."

Hypoglycemia is, without question, a real clinical entity. It does exist, despite the protests of some medical organizations. A substantial amount of evidence indicates that hypoglycemia is caused by an excess intake of refined carbohydrates.[4,5] Although most medical and health organizations, as well as the U.S. government, have recommended that no more than 10% of total caloric intake be derived from refined sugars that are added to foods, the fact is that added sugar accounts for roughly 30% of the total calories consumed by most Americans.[6] The average American consumes over 100 pounds of refined sugar each year. This sugar addiction is part of what is destroying the health of many people.

Hypoglycemia and the Brain

The most critical nutrient for brain function is glucose, or blood sugar. The brain is dependent on glucose as an energy source. When glucose levels are low, as they are in hypoglycemia, the brain does not function properly. Such things as dizziness, headache, blurred vision, blunted mental acuity, emotional instability, confusion, and abnormal behavior may occur. The association between hypoglycemia and impaired mental function is well known. What is not as well known is the effect that hypoglycemia plays in various psychological disorders. For example, despite numerous studies of depressed individuals, which revealed that subjects had a high percentage of abnormal glucose or insulin tolerance, rarely do the physicians of depressed patients look for dietary causes or prescribe dietary therapy.[7,8] There is no explanation for this oversight, especially since dietary therapy (usually the simple elimination of refined carbohydrate from the diet) is occasionally all that is needed for effective therapy of patients with depression due to reactive hypoglycemia.

Aggressive and Criminal Behavior

There is a very strong, yet controversial, link between hypoglycemia and aggressive or criminal behavior. Numerous controlled studies involving psychiatric patients or habitually violent and impulsive criminals have shown that reactive hypoglycemia (as determined by an oral glucose tolerance test) is common in these groups.[9,10] Furthermore, abnormal and sometimes emotionally explosive behavior is often observed during the test. In one study, reactive hypoglycemia was shown to induce fire-setting behavior in arsonists.[11]

A noted criminologist—Stephen J. Schoenthaler, Ph.D.—was intrigued by the evidence presented by another criminologist, Alexander Schauss, in Schauss's landmark work *Diet, Crime, and Delinquency*. Schauss showed that consumption of refined carbohydrates could be linked to criminal and aggressive behavior. In an effort to evaluate the effect of dietary intervention, namely the elimination of refined sugar, on antisocial or aggressive behavior, Schoenthaler conducted several large studies that would eventually involve over 6,000 inmates in 10 penal institutions in three states.[9,12,13]

In Schoenthaler's first study, 174 incarcerated juvenile delinquents were placed on a sugar-restricted diet while another 102 offenders were placed on a control diet.[12] During this two-year study the number of incidents of antisocial behavior decreased by 45%. The most significant changes were in the reduction of assaults (83%), theft (77%), horseplay (65%), and refusal to obey an order (55%). Antisocial behavior changed the most in those charged with assault, robbery, rape, aggravated assault, auto theft, vandalism, child molestation, arson, and possession of a deadly weapon.

In the largest study, 3,999 incarcerated juveniles were studied over a period of two years.[13] This study limited the number of dietary revisions to fruit juices (which replaced sugary soft drinks) and nonrefined carbohydrate snacks (which replaced high-sugar snacks). For example, in the study a serving of popcorn replaced a candy bar. When the behavior of the 1,121 juveniles on the sugar-restricted diet was compared to that of the 884 juveniles on the control diet, significant differences became apparent. In the group with the sugar-restricted diet, suicide attempts were reduced by 100%, the need for restraints to prevent self-injury was reduced by 75%, disruptive behavior was reduced by 42%, and assaults and fights were reduced by 25%. Interestingly, the dietary changes did not seem to affect the behavior of female subjects. This lack of effect may indicate that men may react to hypoglycemia in a different manner than women. From an anthropological and evolutionary view, this makes sense. Low blood sugar levels were undoubtedly an internal signal for men to hunt for food.

The link between hypoglycemia and aggressive behavior extends to men without a history of criminal activity. In one study, a glucose tolerance test was given to a group of men who did not have a history of aggressive behavior or hypoglycemia.[9] This study showed a significant correlation between the tendency to become mildly hypoglycemic and scores on questionnaires used to measure aggression. These results indicate that aggressiveness often coincides with hypoglycemia.

Premenstrual Syndrome

Premenstrual syndrome (PMS) is a recurrent condition of women. It is characterized by troublesome, yet often ill-defined symptoms that usually appear 7 to 14 days before menstruation. The syndrome affects about one-third of women between 30 to 40 years of age, about 10% of whom may have a significantly debilitating form.

One of the leading authorities on PMS is Guy Abraham, M.D. In an attempt to clarify the different forms of PMS, Dr. Abraham subdivided PMS into four distinct subgroups: A, C, D, and H.[14] Each subgroup is linked to specific symptoms, hormonal patterns, and metabolic abnormalities.

PMS-C is associated with increased appetite, a craving for sweets, headache, fatigue, fainting spells, and heart palpitations. When Dr. Abraham gave glucose tolerance tests to PMS-C patients 5 to 10 days before their menses, the results typically implied excessive secretion of insulin in response to sugar consumption. This excessive secretion appears to be hormonally regulated, but other factors may also be involved.[15] During other parts of the menstrual cycle, these women's GTT results were normal.[14] Salt (sodium chloride) enhances insulin response to sugar ingestion, and decreased magnesium levels in the pancreas can result in increased secretion of insulin in response to glucose.

Regardless of the reason, women with PMS-C appear to be extremely sensitive to hypoglycemia.

Migraine Headaches

Migraine headaches are caused by excessive dilation (expansion) of blood vessels in the head. A migraine headache is characterized by a sharp throbbing pain. Migraines are a surprisingly common disorder, affecting 15% to 20% of men and 25% to 30% of women. More than half of migraine patients have a family history of the illness. Hypoglycemia has been shown to be a common precipitating factor in migraine headaches since 1933.[16]

Several studies have found that eliminating refined sugar from the diet of migraine sufferers with confirmed hypoglycemia brings about tremendous improvements. In one study of 48 migraine sufferers with reactive hypoglycemia, 27 (56%) showed greater than 75% improvement in symptoms, 17 (35%) showed greater than 50% improvement, and four (8%) showed greater than 25% improvement.[17]

Atherosclerosis, Angina, and Intermittent Claudication

Atherosclerosis refers to the hardening of the artery walls due to a buildup of plaque containing cholesterol, fatty material, and cellular debris. Because atherosclerosis leads to heart disease and stroke, it is responsible for at least 43% of all deaths in the United States. Atherosclerosis is largely a disease of diet and lifestyle. Lowering the level of LDL cholesterol is the foremost goal in the prevention of atherosclerosis, but preventing hypoglycemia is also important.

There is substantial evidence that reactive hypoglycemia due to a high intake of refined sugar is a significant factor in the development of atherosclerosis.[18] Although a high sugar intake leads to elevations in triglyceride and cholesterol levels, the real culprit may be the elevation of insulin. Remember: In most cases of reactive hypoglycemia, a rapid rise in blood sugar due to sugar consumption causes the body to excrete excessive amounts of insulin. Abnormal results on glucose tolerance tests and elevations in insulin secretion are common findings in patients with heart disease.[19]

In addition to playing a role in atherosclerosis, high sugar consumption and reactive hypoglycemia can be a cause of chest pain (angina) and intermittent claudication (a painful type of a cramp that usually occurs in the calf muscle).[20,21] For a discussion of treatment for intermittent claudication, see Chapter 4.

The role of glucose intolerance and cardiovascular disease will be discussed in detail in Chapter 10, which will also discuss syndrome X and natural treatments for high LDL cholesterol and high blood pressure.

Chapter Summary

Hypoglycemia is associated with a long list of symptoms, but its major effects are on brain function and behavior. Depression, mental confusion, emotional instability, aggressive behavior, and a form of PMS have all been linked to hypoglycemia. Hypoglycemia is also viewed as playing a role in migraine headaches and atherosclerosis.

5

Carbohydrates, the Glycemic Index, and Fiber

The intake of dietary carbohydrates and fiber can affect the level of blood sugar. This chapter will examine carbohydrates in detail and discuss the glycemic index, one means of gauging the effect of specific carbohydrates on blood sugar. This chapter will also explain how dietary fiber affects diabetes and hypoglycemia.

The Importance of Carbohydrates

Dietary carbohydrates play a central role in the cause, prevention, and treatment of both diabetes and hypoglycemia. Carbohydrates are required to provide us with the energy we need for body functions. There are two groups of carbohydrates, simple and complex.

Simple Carbohydrates

Simple carbohydrates, or sugars, are quickly absorbed by the body and provide a ready source of energy. Many believe that the assortment of natural simple sugars in fruits and vegetables have an advantage over sucrose (white sugar) and other refined sugars: The natural sugars are accompanied in foods by a wide range of nutrients that aid in the utilization of the sugars. Problems with carbohydrates begin when they are refined and stripped of these nutrients. Virtually all the vitamin content has been removed from breakfast cereals, white sugar, and the breads and pastries made with white sugar.

As stated earlier, when high-sugar foods are eaten alone, the blood sugar level rises quickly, producing a strain on blood sugar control. Eating foods high in simple sugars can be harmful to blood sugar control—especially if you are hypoglycemic or diabetic. Read food labels carefully for clues about sugar content. If the words "sucrose, glucose, maltose, lactose, fructose, corn syrup," or "white grape juice concentrate" appear on the label, extra sugar has been added. Currently, more than half the carbohydrates being consumed are in the form of sugars that have been added to foods as sweetening agents.

Types of Simple Sugars   Simple sugars are either monosaccharides (composed of one sugar molecule) or disaccharides (composed of two sugar molecules). The principal monosaccharides that occur in foods are glucose and fructose. The major disaccharides are sucrose (white sugar), which is composed of one molecule of glucose and one molecule of fructose; maltose, composed of glucose and glucose; and lactose, composed of glucose and galactose.

Glucose is not particularly sweet tasting compared to fructose and sucrose. It is found in abundant amounts in fruits, honey, sweet corn, and most root vegetables. Glucose is also the primary repeating sugar unit of most complex carbohydrates.

Fructose, or fruit sugar, is the primary carbohydrate in many fruits, maple syrup, and honey. Fructose is very sweet

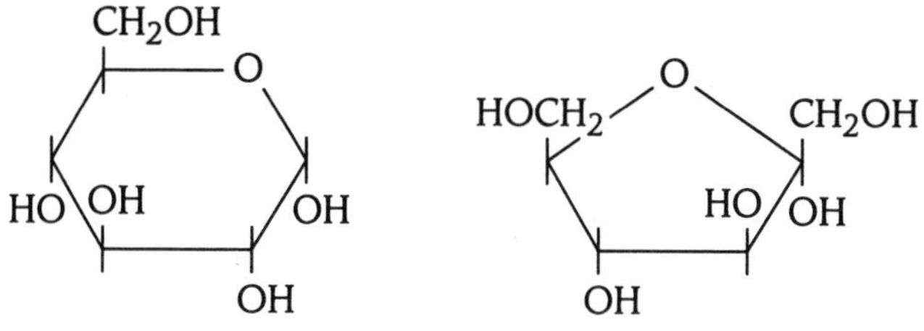

Glucose   Fructose

Figure 5.1   Chemical structures of glucose and fructose

and is roughly 1½ times sweeter than sucrose (white sugar). Although fructose has the same chemical formula as glucose ($C_6H_{12}O_6$), its structure (shape) is quite different, as Figure 5.1 shows. To be utilized by the body, the liver must convert fructose to glucose.

Complex Carbohydrates

Complex carbohydrates, or starches, are composed of many simple sugars joined together by chemical bonds. The body breaks down complex carbohydrates into simple sugars gradually, which leads to a relatively stable blood sugar level. More and more research is indicating that complex carbohydrates should form a major part of the diet. Vegetables, legumes, and grains are excellent sources of complex carbohydrates.

The Effects of Fructose on Blood Sugar

Many physicians have recommended that individuals with diabetes or hypoglycemia avoid fruits and fructose. However, recent research challenges this recommendation.

Fructose does not cause a rapid rise in the blood sugar level. Because fructose must be changed to glucose in the liver to be utilized by the body, the blood glucose level does not rise as rapidly after fructose consumption as it does after consumption of other simple sugars. For example, the ingestion of sucrose results in an immediate elevation of blood sugar. While most diabetics and hypoglycemics cannot tolerate sucrose, most can tolerate moderate amounts of fruits and fructose, without loss of blood sugar control. In fact, fructose and fruits are not only much better tolerated than white bread and other refined carbohydrates, they produce elevations in the blood sugar level that are less pronounced than those caused by most sources of complex carbohydrates (starch).[1,2] As a bonus, when fed to non–insulin dependent diabetics over four weeks, fructose has actually been shown to enhance the sensitivity to insulin by 34%.[1]

Regular fruit consumption may also help control sugar cravings, decrease the amount of calories and fat consumed, and promote weight loss in overweight individuals. In contrast, studies have shown aspartame (Nutrasweet), glucose, and sucrose to increase the appetite. Typically, in such studies subjects eat or drink something containing fructose or an equal amount of some other sweetener. Then, 30 minutes to 2½ hours later, they are invited to consume as much food as they desire at a dinner buffet. The studies are designed in a double-blind fashion so that neither observers nor participants know who has been given what. Consistently, subjects receiving the fructose-sweetened food or drink eat substantially fewer calories and fat than those receiving aspartame, sucrose, or glucose.[3-5]

Since fruits contain fructose in a natural form, consuming a serving of fruit or fruit juice at least 30 minutes before dinner may result in significantly fewer calories consumed. When fewer calories are consumed, weight loss is much easier to achieve. Fruits make excellent between-meal snacks that help stabilize blood sugar.

Fruits are also excellent sources of numerous health-promoting substances, including vitamin C, carotenes, pectin and other fibers, flavonoids, and polyphenols such as ellagic acid. Regular fruit consumption has been shown to offer significant protection against many chronic degenerative diseases including cancer, heart disease, cataracts, and stroke.[6] Given the important nutritional qualities of fruits, it simply doesn't make sense to avoid eating them.

The Glycemic Index

David Jenkins developed the glycemic index in 1981 to express the rise of blood glucose after eating a particular food.[7] The standard value of 100 is based on the rise caused by the ingestion of glucose. The glycemic index ranges from about 20, for fructose and whole barley, to about 98, for a baked potato. The insulin response to carbohydrate-containing foods is similar to the rise in blood sugar. Table 5.1 shows the glycemic index values of many common foods.[8]

The glycemic index is used as a guideline for making dietary recommendations for people with either diabetes or hypoglycemia. Basically, people with blood sugar problems should avoid foods with high values and choose carbohydrate-containing foods, which have lower values. However, the glycemic index should not be the only dietary guideline. For example, although high-fat foods, such as ice cream and sausage, may have a low glycemic index (because a diet high in fat has been shown to impair glucose tolerance), these foods are not wise food choices for people with hypoglycemia or diabetes.

The Importance of Fiber

Population studies, as well as clinical and experimental data, show diabetes to be one of the diseases most clearly related

Table 5.1   Glycemic Index Values for Some Common Foods

Sugars		Grains *(continued)*	
Fructose	20	Bread, white	69
Glucose	100	Bread, whole grain	72
Honey	75	Corn	59
Maltose	105	Cornflakes	80
Sucrose	60	Oatmeal	49
Fruits		Pasta	45
Apples	39	Rice	70
Bananas	62	Rice, puffed	95
Orange juice	46	Wheat cereal	67
Oranges	40		
Raisins	64	*Legumes*	
		Beans	31
Vegetables		Lentils	29
Beets	64	Peas	39
Carrot, cooked	36		
Carrot, raw	31	*Other foods*	
Potato, baked	98	Ice cream	36
Potato (new), boiled	70	Milk	34
Grains		Nuts	13
Bran cereal	51	Sausages	28

to inadequate dietary fiber intake.[6,9] The results indicate that, while the intake of refined sugars should be curtailed, the intake of complex carbohydrate sources that are rich in fiber should be increased.

The term *dietary fiber* refers to components of the plant cell wall as well as the indigestible residues from plant foods. Different types of fiber possess different actions. The type of fiber that exerts the most beneficial effects on blood sugar control are the water-soluble forms. Included in this class are hemicelluloses, mucilages, gums, and pectin substances. These types of fiber are capable of slowing down the digestion and absorption of carbohydrates, thereby preventing rapid rises in blood sugar; increasing the sensitivity of tissues to insulin, thereby preventing the excessive secretion of insulin; and improving the uptake of glucose by the liver and other tissues, thereby preventing a sustained elevation of blood sugar.

Fortunately, the majority of fiber in the walls of most plant cells is water soluble. Particularly good sources of water-soluble fiber are legumes (beans), oat bran, nuts, seeds, the seed husks of psyllium, pears, apples, and most vegetables (see Table 5.2). The important thing is to consume a large amount of plant foods to obtain adequate levels of dietary fiber. A daily intake of 50 grams is a healthful goal.

Table 5.2 Dietary Fiber Content of Selected Foods

Food	Serving	Calories	Grams of Fiber
Fruits			
Apple (with skin)	1 medium	81	3.5
Banana	1 medium	105	2.4
Cantaloupe	¼ melon	30	1.0
Cherries, sweet	10	49	1.2
Grapefruit	½ medium	38	1.6
Orange	1 medium	62	2.6
Peach (with skin)	1	37	1.9
Pear (with skin)	½ large	61	3.1
Prunes	3	60	3.0
Raisins	¼ cup	106	3.1
Raspberries	½ cup	35	3.1
Strawberries	1 cup	45	3.0
Vegetables, raw			
Bean sprouts	½ cup	13	1.5
Celery, diced	½ cup	10	1.1
Cucumber	½ cup	8	0.4
Lettuce	1 cup	10	0.9
Mushrooms	½ cup	10	1.5
Pepper, green	½ cup	9	0.5
Spinach	1 cup	8	1.2
Tomato	1 medium	20	1.5

Table 5.2   (continued)

Food	Serving	Calories	Grams of Fiber
Vegetables, cooked			
Asparagus, cut	1 cup	30	2.0
Beans, green	1 cup	32	3.2
Broccoli	1 cup	40	4.4
Brussels sprouts	1 cup	56	4.6
Cabbage, red	1 cup	30	2.8
Carrots	1 cup	48	4.6
Cauliflower	1 cup	28	2.2
Corn	½ cup	87	2.9
Kale	1 cup	44	2.8
Parsnip	1 cup	102	5.4
Potato (with skin)	1 medium	106	2.5
Potato (without skin)	1 medium	97	1.4
Spinach	1 cup	42	4.2
Sweet potato	1 medium	160	3.4
Zucchini	1 cup	22	3.6
Legumes			
Baked beans	½ cup	155	8.8
Dried peas, cooked	½ cup	115	4.7
Kidney beans, cooked	½ cup	110	7.3
Lima beans, cooked	½ cup	64	4.5
Lentils, cooked	½ cup	97	3.7
Navy beans, cooked	½ cup	112	6.0
Rice, breads, pastas			
Bran muffins	1 muffin	104	2.5
Bread, white	1 slice	78	0.4
Bread, whole wheat	1 slice	61	1.4
Crisp bread, rye	2 crackers	50	2.0
Rice, brown, cooked	½ cup	97	1.0
Rice, white, cooked	½ cup	82	0.2
Spaghetti, regular, cooked	½ cup	155	1.1

Table 5.2   (continued)

Food	Serving	Calories	Grams of Fiber
Spaghetti, whole wheat, cooked	½ cup	155	3.9
Breakfast cereals			
All-Bran	⅓ cup	71	8.5
Bran Chex	⅔ cup	91	4.6
Corn Bran	⅔ cup	98	5.4
Cornflakes	1¼ cups	110	0.3
Grape-Nuts	¼ cup	101	1.4
Oatmeal	¾ cup	108	1.6
Raisin Bran type	⅔ cup	115	4.0
Shredded Wheat	⅔ cup	102	2.6
Nuts			
Almonds	10 nuts	79	1.1
Filberts	10 nuts	54	0.8
Peanuts	10 nuts	105	1.4

Chapter Summary

Dietary carbohydrates are divided into two major categories: simple and complex. Different carbohydrates will produce different effects on the blood sugar level. The glycemic index expresses the rise of blood glucose after eating a particular food. The glycemic index is used as a guideline for dietary recommendations for people with either diabetes or hypoglycemia. People with blood sugar problems should avoid foods with high glycemic index values and choose carbohydrate-containing foods which have lower values. Dietary fiber exerts many beneficial effects in the prevention, control, and treatment of blood sugar disorders.

6

Dietary Guidelines and Menu Suggestions

D iet is fundamental to the successful treatment of diabetes, whether it be type I or II, and hypoglycemia. Although there are several commonly recommended diets to manage these diseases, the one this chapter will describe is based on the diet popularized by Dr. James Anderson.[1] The diet is high in cereal grains, legumes, and root vegetables, and it restricts simple sugar and fat intake. It is called the high complex-carbohydrate, high-fiber diet, or HCF diet.

The scientific literature validates the importance of a high complex-carbohydrate, high-fiber diet in the treatment of diabetes and hypoglycemia. Such a diet is also low in fat. The link between fat intake and diabetes is nearly as strong as the link between refined sugar intake and diabetes. It is interesting to note that, before 1955, recommendations to diabetics included the suggestion that they derive the majority of their calories from fat. Although the resulting diets provided short-term benefits in glucose control, the long-term consequences were extremely detrimental and even fatal. A diet high in fat actually leads to insulin insensitivity and greatly increases the risk of atherosclerosis, the buildup of cholesterol-containing plaque in medium-sized and large arteries.[1]

The positive effects of the HCF diet for diabetics are many. They include:

- Reduction of abnormally high after-meal blood sugar
- Increased sensitivity of tissue to insulin
- Reduction of low-density lipoproteins (LDLs), cholesterol that increases the risk of atherosclerosis
- Increase of high-density lipoproteins (HDLs), cholesterol that lowers the danger of atherosclerosis
- Reduction of triglycerides (stored fat) and progressive weight reduction

Compared to other diets, even the one recommended by the American Diabetes Association, the HCF diet has proved superior. For example, when type I diabetics who have followed the HCF diet resume the diet recommended by the American Diabetes Association, their insulin requirements return to prior levels.[2] The HCF diet has also been shown to be extremely effective in treating hypoglycemia.[3]

Anderson outlined two HCF diets: one for the initial treatment of the hospitalized patient and one for home use, or health maintenance. In the hospital version, the caloric intake consists of 70% to 75% complex carbohydrates, 15% to 20% protein, and only 5% to 10% fat. The total fiber content is almost 100 grams per day. The caloric intake of the maintenance diet consists of 55% to 60% complex carbohydrates, 20% protein, and 20% to 25% fat. The total fiber content is still almost 100 grams per day.

On the maintenance HCF diet, carbohydrate calories come from grain products (which provide 50% of carbohydrate calories), fruits and vegetables (48%), and skim milk (2%). Protein is provided by fruits and vegetables (50%), grain products (36%), and skim milk and lean meat (14%).

Fat is derived from grain products (60%), fruits and vegetables (20%), and skim milk and meat (12%).

The dietary guidelines and menu suggestions given in this chapter will allow the diabetic or hypoglycemic to incorporate complex carbohydrates and fiber along with even more legumes than the HCF diet includes. The caloric and fiber components of the diet you will strive for are as follows.

> Carbohydrates: 65% to 75% of total calories
>
> Fats: 15% to 25% of total calories
>
> Protein: 10% to 15% of total calories
>
> Dietary fiber: At least 50 grams

In essence, by applying what you will learn in this chapter, you can create a version of Anderson's HCF diet that is more healthful than the original. A high-carbohydrate, legume-rich, high-fiber diet has been shown to improve all aspects of diabetes control.[4] Such a diet can result in similar control of hypoglycemia.

Some individuals with diabetes try to increase the fiber content of their diet through supplementation rather than through diet. Although fiber-supplemented diets are beneficial, they are not as effective as those containing fiber from food.[1] The insulin dosages for patients on fiber- supplemented diets can usually be reduced to one-third those for patients on control diets, such as that of the American Diabetes Association. The HCF diet, on the other hand, has led to discontinuation of insulin therapy in approximately 60% of type II patients and significantly reduced doses for the other 40%.

If you are a type I diabetic, be advised: Any change in your diet may result in the need to alter your insulin dosage or schedule. Before you begin the Healthy Exchange System diet or any other, consult with your doctor. Monitor your blood sugar as your doctor advises, and follow his or her instructions about changing your medication.

The Healthy Exchange System

The American Dietetic Association, in conjunction with the American Diabetes Association and other groups, has developed the Exchange System, a convenient tool for the rapid estimation of the calorie, protein, fat, and carbohydrate content of a diet. Originally designed for use in designing dietary recommendations for diabetics, the Exchange System is now used in the design of virtually all therapeutic diets. Unfortunately, the system does not place enough emphasis on the quality of food choices.

The diet this chapter recommends is based on a system of diet design called the Healthy Exchange System. (This system is also the basis for recommendations in *The Healing Power of Foods* and *The Healing Power of Foods Cookbook*. Both books are by Michael T. Murray and published by Prima Publishing, Rocklin, California [1993].) This system is a more healthful version of the Exchange System, because it emphasizes unprocessed, whole foods. The building blocks of the Healthy Exchange System are seven lists, often called exchange lists, two of which (the milk and meat lists) are optional.

List 1	Vegetables
List 2	Fruits
List 3	Breads, cereals, and starchy vegetables
List 4	Legumes
List 5	Fats
List 6	Milk
List 7	Meats, fish, cheese, and eggs

The word *Exchange* in the name *Healthy Exchange System* refers to the fact that any item in a list can be exchanged for any other item in the same list. In other words, you can choose either four medium-sized fresh apricots or 1 medium banana to fulfill a serving requirement for fruit. (Later in this chapter you will examine the seven lists and learn about serving requirements.) The fact that the Healthy Exchange System allows such a wide variety of choices makes it a flexible system that is likely to satisfy your palate as well as your nutritional requirements.

According to the Healthy Exchange System, 90% of carbohydrates ingested should be complex carbohydrates or naturally occurring sugars. Intake of refined carbohydrates and concentrated sugars (including honey, pasteurized fruit juices, and dried fruit, as well as sugar and white flour) should be limited to less than 10% of the total calorie intake.

Using the exchange lists, constructing a diet that meets these recommendations is simple. In addition, the recommendations ensure a high intake of vital whole foods, particularly vegetables, that are rich in nutritional value.

To apply the Healthy Exchange System, you must first determine your caloric needs. These needs vary by sex, body frame size, height, weight, and level of physical activity. In the next three sections, you will learn about the relationship of body weight and weight distribution to diabetes and hypoglycemia. Then you will find out how to determine your own caloric needs.

Body Weight and Blood Sugar

Body weight is a significant factor in blood sugar control. Even in normal individuals, significant weight gain results in carbohydrate intolerance, higher insulin levels, and insulin insensitivity in fat and muscle tissue. The progressive development of insulin insensitivity is believed to be the underlying factor in the development of type II diabetes. Weight loss corrects all these abnormalities and significantly improves the metabolic disturbances of diabetes. In other words, since 90% of people with type II diabetes are obese, the majority of Americans with diabetes could cure themselves simply by achieving their ideal body weight.

Body Fat Distribution: Its Relationship to Diabetes and Hypoglycemia

The distribution of body fat appears to play a significant role in the link between obesity and diabetes. Two basic distribution patterns exist: android and gynecoid obesity. In android obesity, fat is deposited primarily in the upper body—that is, the abdomen. This type of obesity is typically seen in the obese male. A waist measurement that is larger than the hip measurement is diagnostic of this condition. In gynecoid obesity, the fat is distributed primarily in the lower body—the gluteal and femoral areas (around the buttocks and hips). This type of obesity is typically observed in females.

Android obesity can connote a serious metabolic condition. In addition to the association with diabetes, android obesity (whether in a male or female) has been shown to be predictive and strongly related to hypertension and hyperglycemia. When android obesity occurs in a woman, endocrine diseases and gallstone formation often develop.[5-8]

How Many Calories Do You Need?

The first step in determining your caloric needs is to determine the size of your body frame. The next step is to determine ideal body weight and calculate the number of calories necessary to sustain that weight.

Determining Frame Size

Extend your arm and bend the forearm upward at a 90-degree angle. Keep the fingers straight and turn the inside of your wrist away from your body. Place the thumb and index finger of your other hand on the two prominent bones on either side of your elbow. Measure the space between your fingers with a tape measure. Two lists follow, one for men and one for women. Using whichever is appropriate, find your height in the left column. Compare the measurement of the breadth of your elbow with the elbow measurement beside your height. The elbow breadths listed are for medium-framed individuals. If the measurement of your elbow is smaller than the range cited in the table, you have a small frame; if it is larger, you have a large frame.

Height in 1″ Heels	Elbow Breadth
Men	
5′2″– 5′3″	$2^1/_2″ -2^7/_8″$
5′4″–5′7″	$2^5/_8″ -2^7/_8″$
5′8″–5′11″	$2^3/_4″ -3″$
6′0″–6′3″	$2^3/_4″ -3^1/_8″$
6′4″	$2^7/_8″ -3^1/_4″$
Women	
4′10″–5′3″	$2^1/_4″ -2^1/_2″$
5′4″–5′11″	$2^3/_8″ -2^5/_8″$
6′0″	$2^1/_2″ -2^3/_4″$

Now that you know the size of your body frame, you can determine the body weight appropriate for it.

Determining Ideal Body Weight

The most popular tables of "desirable" weight are those provided by the Metropolitan Life Insurance Company (Table 6.1). The most recent edition of these tables, published

Table 6.1   1983 Metropolitan Life Insurance Tables of Ideal Body Weight*

Height	Small Frame	Weight (pounds) Medium Frame	Large Frame
Men			
5'2"	128–134	131–141	138–150
5'3"	130–136	133–143	140–153
5'4"	132–138	135–145	142–156
5'5"	134–140	137–148	144–160
5'6"	136–142	139–151	146–164
5'7"	138–145	142–154	149–168
5'8"	140–148	145–157	152–172
5'9"	142–151	148–160	155–176
5'10"	144–154	151–163	158–180
5'11"	146–157	154–166	161–184
6'0"	149–160	157–170	164–188
6'1"	152–164	160–174	168–192
6'2"	155–168	164–178	172–197
6'3"	158–172	167–182	176–202
6'4"	162–176	171–187	181–207
Women			
4'10"	102–111	109–121	118–131
4'11"	103–113	111–123	120–134
5'0"	104–115	113–126	122–137
5'1"	106–118	115–129	125–140
5'2"	108–121	118–132	128–143
5'3"	111–124	121–135	131–147
5'4"	114–127	124–138	134–151
5'5"	117–130	127–141	137–155
5'6"	120–133	130–144	140–159
5'7"	123–136	133–147	143–163
5'8"	126–139	136–150	146–167
5'9"	129–142	139–153	149–170
5'10"	132–145	142–156	152–173
5'11"	135–148	145–159	155–176
6'0"	138–151	148–162	158–179

*Weights cited are, in pounds, for adults age 25–59 years, based on lowest mortality. Weight is cited according to frame size in indoor clothing (5 pounds for men and 3 pounds for women), wearing shoes with 1" heels.

in 1983, gives weight ranges for men and women, in 1-inch increments of height, for three body frame sizes. The next step in determining your daily caloric needs is to make a calculation involving weight and activity level.

Factoring in Your Activity Level

Convert your ideal weight in pounds to kilograms by multiplying it by 0.4536. Next choose, from the list that follows, the activity level that best describes your activity level.

Little physical activity	30 calories
Light physical activity	35 calories
Moderate physical activity	40 calories
Heavy physical activity	45 calories

Make a note of the number of calories cited after the level that you chose. You will use this number in the equation that calculates the number of calories you need each day. The equation follows.

In the formula, insert the value for your own weight, in kilograms, and the number of calories associated with your level of activity. Do the multiplication required to find approximate daily caloric requirements.

Weight (in kg)	×	Number of calories for activity level	=	Approximate daily calorie requirements
_____	×	_____	=	_____

The Diets of the Healthy Exchange System

As you recall, the Healthy Exchange System defines seven lists—five mandatory and two optional—that categorize foods according to broad groups. The diets in the Healthy Exchange System define the number of servings you should eat from the lists. The diets provide total daily calories in the range of 1,000 to 3,000 calories, in increments of 500 calories. The system offers two diets at each level: one for the vegan, or person who does not consume meat or dairy products, and one for the omnivore, or person who eats animal and vegetable substances.

As an example of one of the diets, study the 1,500 vegan diet, which follows.

1,500-Calorie Vegan Diet

List 1 (vegetables):	5 servings
List 2 (fruits):	2 servings
List 3 (breads, cereals, and starchy vegetables):	9 servings
List 4 (legumes):	2½ servings
List 5 (fats):	4 servings

This diet would result in an intake of approximately 1,500 calories, of which 67% are derived from complex carbohydrates (cereals, fruits, and vegetables) and naturally occurring sugars, 18% from fats, and 15% from proteins. The protein intake is entirely from plant sources, but still provides approximately 55 grams, an amount well above the recommended daily allowance of protein intake for someone requiring 1,500 calories. At least one-half of the fat servings should be from nuts, seeds, and other whole foods from list 5, the fat exchange list. The dietary fiber intake would be 31 to 74.5 grams. The list that follows summarizes this information.

Percentage of calories as carbohydrates: 67%

Percentage of calories as fats: 18%

Percentage of calories as protein: 15%

Protein content: 55 grams

Dietary fiber content: 31 to 74.5 grams

The preceding list—which shows percentages, protein content, and dietary fiber—is important because it allows you to compare the proportions of each Healthy Exchange System diet with the proportions of the "ideal" diet, which were cited on page 47. The remainder of this section presents the other diets of the Healthy Exchange System. Find the one that provides the calorie intake appropriate for you.

In the next section, you will examine each list in detail and learn how to use the lists to meet the requirements of the diet you have chosen.

1,500-Calorie Omnivore Diet

List 1 (vegetables):	5 servings
List 2 (fruits):	2½ servings
List 3 (breads, cereals, and starchy vegetables):	6 servings
List 4 (legumes):	1 serving
List 5 (fats):	5 servings
List 6 (milk):	1 serving
List 7 (meats, fish, cheese, and eggs):	2 servings

Percentage of calories as carbohydrates: 67%
Percentage of calories as fats: 18%
Percentage of calories as protein: 15%
Protein content: 61 grams (75% from plant sources)
Dietary fiber content: 19.5 to 53.5 grams

2,000-Calorie Vegan Diet

List 1 (vegetables):	5½ servings
List 2 (fruits):	2 servings
List 3 (breads, cereals, and starchy vegetables):	11 servings

List 4 (legumes):   5 servings
List 5 (fats):   8 servings
  Percentage of calories as carbohydrates: 67%
  Percentage of calories as fats: 18%
  Percentage of calories as protein: 15%
  Protein content: 79 grams
  Dietary fiber content: 48.5 to 101.5 grams

2,000-Calorie Omnivore Diet
List 1 (vegetables):   5 servings
List 2 (fruits):   2½ servings
List 3 (breads, cereals, and starchy
vegetables):   13 servings
List 4 (legumes):   2 servings
List 5 (fats):   7 servings
List 6 (milk):   1 serving
List 7 (meats, fish, cheese, and eggs):   2 servings
  Percentage of calories as carbohydrates: 66%
  Percentage of calories as fats: 19%
  Percentage of calories as protein: 15%
  Protein content: 78 grams (72% from plant sources)
  Dietary fiber content: 32.5 to 88.5 grams

2,500-Calorie Vegan Diet
List 1 (vegetables):   8 servings
List 2 (fruits):   3 servings
List 3 (breads, cereals, and starchy
vegetables):   17 servings
List 4 (legumes):   5 servings
List 5 (fats):   8 servings

Percentage of calories as carbohydrates: 69%
Percentage of calories as fats: 15%
Percentage of calories as protein: 16%
Protein content: 101 grams
Dietary fiber content: 33 to 121 grams

2,500-Calorie Omnivore Diet

List 1 (vegetables):	8 servings
List 2 (fruits):	3½ servings
List 3 (breads, cereals, and starchy vegetables):	17 servings
List 4 (legumes):	2 servings
List 5 (fats):	8 servings
List 6 (milk):	1 serving
List 7 (meats, fish, cheese, and eggs):	3 servings

Percentage of calories as carbohydrates: 66%
Percentage of calories as fats: 18%
Percentage of calories as protein: 16%
Protein content: 102 grams (80% from plant sources)
Dietary fiber content: 40.5 to 116.5 grams

3,000-Calorie Vegan Diet

List 1 (vegetables):	10 servings
List 2 (fruits):	4 servings
List 3 (breads, cereals, and starchy vegetables):	17 servings
List 4 (legumes):	6 servings
List 5 (fats):	10 servings

Percentage of calories as carbohydrates: 70%
Percentage of calories as fats: 16%

Percentage of calories as protein: 14%
Protein content: 116 grams
Dietary fiber content: 50 to 84 grams

3,000-Calorie Omnivore Diet

List 1 (vegetables):	10 servings
List 2 (fruits):	3 servings
List 3 (breads, cereals, and starchy vegetables):	20 servings
List 4 (legumes):	2 servings
List 5 (fats):	10 servings
List 6 (milk):	1 serving
List 7 (meats, fish, cheese, and eggs):	3 servings

Percentage of calories as carbohydrates: 67%
Percentage of calories as fats: 18%
Percentage of calories as protein: 15%
Protein content: 116 grams (81% from plant sources)
Dietary fiber content: 45 to 133 grams

Note: You can use these diets as the basis for calculating other diets of specific calorie amounts. For example, for a 4,000-calorie diet, add the 2,500-calorie diet to the 1,500-calorie diet. For a 1,000-calorie diet, divide the 2,000-calorie diet in half.

The Healthy Exchange Lists

In this part of the chapter, you will examine each exchange list in the Healthy Exchange System. You will learn about the general characteristics of each category of food and how individual foods can benefit you or be detrimental to nutrition. This is the part of the chapter in which each exchange list appears. From these lists, each day, you will choose foods to meet the serving requirements defined by your diet.

List 1: Vegetables

Vegetables provide the broadest range of nutrients of any food class. They are rich sources of vitamins, minerals, carbohydrates, and protein. The little fat they contain is in the form of essential fatty acids. Vegetables provide high quantities of other valuable health-promoting substances, especially carotene (a substance the body can convert into vitamin A) and fiber. In Latin, the word *vegetable* means to enliven or animate. Vegetables give us life. More and more evidence is accumulating that shows that vegetables can prevent as well as treat many diseases.

Vegetables should play a major role in the diet. The National Academy of Science, the U.S. Department of Health and Human Services, and the National Cancer Institute recommend that Americans consume a minimum of three to five servings of vegetables per day.[3] Unfortunately, less than 11% of all Americans achieve this goal.

Vegetables are the richest source of antioxidant compounds, which provide protection against free radicals. Free radicals are highly reactive molecules that bind to and destroy cellular components. Free radicals have been shown to be responsible for many diseases, including the two biggest killers of Americans—heart disease and cancer. Diabetics appear to be especially sensitive to the negative effects of free radicals. For the long-term treatment of diabetes, increasing the intake of dietary antioxidants—carotene, chlorophyll, vitamin C, sulfur-containing compounds, vitamin E, and selenium—is essential. The way to increase the intake of antioxidants is to eat more vegetables.

The best way to consume many vegetables is in their fresh, raw form. In this form, many of the nutrients and health-promoting compounds are provided in much higher concentrations than in processed or cooked forms. Drinking fresh vegetable juice is an excellent way to make sure you are achieving your daily quota of vegetables.

When cooking vegetables, be sure not to overcook them. Overcooking will not only result in the loss of important nutrients, it will alter the flavor. Light steaming, baking, and quick stir-frying are the best ways to cook vegetables. Do not boil vegetables; most of the nutrients will be left in the water. The only exception to this rule is soup making. Since the liquid used for boiling the vegetables is the soup itself, and you will consume the soup, boiling soup vegetables is fine. If fresh vegetables are not available for soup making or any other purpose, frozen vegetables are preferred over their canned counterparts.

Although pickled vegetables are quite popular, they may not be healthful choices. Not only are they high in salt, they may also be high in cancer-causing compounds. Several population studies in China have suggested an association between consumption of pickled vegetables and cancer of the esophagus.[9] The harmful substances in pickled vegetables are N-nitroso compounds. Once ingested, these compounds can form potent cancer-causing nitrosamines.

Vegetables are fantastic "diet" foods because they are very high in nutritional value but low in calories. In the list that follows you will notice there is a category of "free" vegetables. These vegetables are termed free because you can eat them in any amount desired; the calories they contain will be offset by the number of calories your body will burn to digest them. If you are trying to lose weight, these foods are especially valuable because they will help to keep you feeling satisfied between meals.

Vegetables

Measured-serving vegetables

The list that follows shows the vegetables to use for 1 vegetable serving. Unless otherwise noted, 1 serving consists of 1 cup cooked vegetable or fresh vegetable juice or 2 cups raw vegetable. Notice that starchy vegetables, such as potatoes and yams, are included in list 3 (breads, cereals, and starchy vegetables).

Artichoke (1 medium)
Asparagus
Bean sprouts
Beets
Broccoli
Brussels sprouts
Carrots
Cauliflower
Eggplant
Greens
    Beet
    Chard
    Collard
    Dandelion
    Kale
    Mustard
    Spinach
    Turnip
Mushrooms
Okra
Onions
Rhubarb
Rutabaga
Sauerkraut
String beans, green or yellow
Summer squash
Tomatoes, tomato juice, vegetable juice cocktail
Zucchini

Free vegetables

The following vegetables may be used as often as desired. They are especially healthful in their raw form.

Alfalfa sprouts

Bell peppers

Bok choy

Cabbage

Celery

Chicory

Chinese cabbage

Cucumber

Endive

Escarole

Lettuce

Parsley

Radishes

Spinach

Turnips

Watercress

List 2: Fruits

Fruits are a rich source of many beneficial compounds. Regular fruit consumption has been shown to offer significant protection against many chronic degenerative diseases. Among them are cancer, heart disease, cataracts, and stroke. Fruits make excellent snacks, because they contain fructose, or fruit sugar. Because fructose is sweet, it tends to satisfy the snacker and serve as a psychological treat. Fructose is not as disruptive to metabolism as some other sugars, however. The bloodstream absorbs fructose slowly, thereby allowing the body time to utilize it. Fruits are also excellent sources of vitamins and minerals as well as health-promoting fiber compounds. However, fruits are not as nutritious as vegetables, because they tend to be higher in calories. That is why vegetables are favored over fruits in weight-loss plans and healthful diets. Because they contain so much vitamin C and fiber and so many antioxidants and flavonoids (see Chapter 7), fruits may offer significant benefit in the treatment of diabetes as well as the prevention of diabetic complications.

In regard to its effect on diabetes, the tropical fruit guava has been the focus of much discussion. According to Chinese folklore, guava can cause remarkable benefits for diabetics. To verify this, researchers in Taiwan investigated the effect of guava juice in normal and diabetic animals and humans. The effects of giving roughly 3 ounces of guava juice was the same in both normal and diabetic human volunteers: Blood sugar was reduced for up to 3 hours. In the diabetic individuals studied, 3 ounces of guava juice caused the mean value of blood glucose to fall from 214 milligrams per deciliter to 165 milligrams per deciliter.[10]

These results alone appear to confirm the benefits of guava for diabetics, but there is more. In a study published in the *American Journal of Cardiology,* 120 subjects were divided into two groups. Group A was instructed to eat one guava (roughly 3½ ounces) each day before a meal.[11] Group B served as the control group; Group B participants were asked to maintain their usual dietary practices.

Group A, the guava-eating group, showed a 9.9% reduction in total blood cholesterol, a 7.7% reduction in triglycerides, and an 8% increase in high-density lipoprotein (HDL) cholesterol. Group A also had a significant decrease in blood pressure (an average drop of 9/8 millimeters of mercury). Guava is a good source of soluble fiber, vitamin C, and potassium. These nutrients alone have been shown to produce effects similar to those enjoyed by Group A, but the benefit of guava appears to go beyond the effects of these nutrients.

Since guava is not always available in the United States, Americans may have to turn to grapefruit. Grapefruit may be a suitable alternative to guava. Researchers at the University of Florida, who were led by Dr. James Cerda, have studied grapefruit pectin extensively since 1973. The researchers focused on the cholesterol-lowering effects of grapefruit pectin. The edible portion of a grapefruit contains approximately 3.9% pectin. Since most of the cholesterol-lowering studies used 15 grams of grapefruit pectin to produce a 10% drop in cholesterol, you would need to eat about two whole grapefruits to achieve a similar pectin level. Grapefruit or guava—it doesn't seem to matter. Both are capable of reducing cholesterol by about 10%. Because every 1% drop in cholesterol means a 2% drop in the risk of heart disease, the act of eating two grapefruit or guava per day can lower the risk of heart disease by 20%. This benefit is significant for diabetics, because diabetes causes such a tremendous increase in the risk of heart disease.

If you are a diabetic, monitor your blood glucose level after drinking guava juice, grapefruit juice, or any fruit juice. If the level is higher than 200 milligrams of glucose per deciliter or less than 80 milligrams of glucose per deciliter, consult your doctor. He or she may advise that you change the dosage of your medication.

The Healthy Exchange list for fruit follows. You will note that the list includes a few items made from processed fruit—jams, jellies, and preserves—and a few items that are not fruit at all—honey and sugar. Do not eat more than one serving per day of these processed products.

Fruits

Fresh fruit and fruit-based items
Each of the following items equals 1 serving.

Fresh juice, 1 cup (8 ounces)*
Pasteurized juice, ⅔ cup

Apple, 1 large
Applesauce (unsweetened), 1 cup
Apricots, dried, 8 halves
Apricots, fresh, 4 medium
Banana, 1 medium
Berries
    Blackberries, 1 cup
    Blueberries, 1 cup
    Cranberries, 1 cup
    Raspberries, 1 cup
    Strawberries, 1½ cups
Cherries, 20 large
Dates, 4
Figs, dried, 2
Figs, fresh, 2
Grapefruit, 1
Grapes, 20
Mango, 1 small
Melons
    Cantaloupe, ½ small
    Honeydew, ¼ medium
    Watermelon, 2 cups
Nectarines, 2 small
Orange, 1 large
Papaya, 1½ cups
Peaches, 2 medium
Persimmons, 2 medium
Pineapple, 1 cup
Plums, 4 medium
Prune juice, 1/2 cup
Prunes, 4 medium

Raisins, 4 tablespoons

Tangerines, 2 medium

Processed fruit and other products
Eat no more than 1 serving of the following "fruit" foods per day.

Honey, 1 tablespoon

Jams, jellies, preserves, 1 tablespoon

Sugar, 1 tablespoon

*Although 1 cup of most juices equals 1 serving, prune juice is an exception; consult the alphabetized portion of the list.

List 3: Breads, Cereals, and Starchy Vegetables

Breads, cereals, and starchy vegetables are classified as complex carbohydrates. Chemically, complex carbohydrates are made up of long chains of simple carbohydrates or sugars. This means the human body has to digest, or break down, the large sugar chains into simple sugars. Therefore, the sugar from complex carbohydrates enters the bloodstream relatively slowly. This means a relatively stable blood sugar level and appetite.

Complex carbohydrates—breads, cereals, and starchy vegetables—are higher in fiber and nutrients and lower in calories than simple-sugar items such as cakes and candies. Choose whole-grain products (whole-grain bread, whole-grain flour products, brown rice, and the like) over their processed counterparts (white bread, white-flour products, white rice, and so on). Whole grains are a major source of complex carbohydrates, dietary fiber, minerals, and B vitamins. The protein content and quality of whole grains is greater than that of refined grains. Diets rich in whole grains have been shown to guard against chronic degenerative diseases. Whole-grain diets are especially significant in the prevention of cancer, heart disease, diabetes, varicose veins, and diseases of the colon (colon cancer; inflammatory bowel disease, such as diverticulitis; and hemorrhoids).[3] Whole grains can be used as breakfast cereals, side dishes, or casseroles or as part of the entrée. Whole-grain recipes follow, later in this chapter. *The Healing Power of Foods Cookbook* also contains whole-grain recipes. Note that some of the prepared foods included in the list of breads, cereals, and starchy vegetables constitute more than 1 serving.

Breads, Cereals, and Starchy Vegetables
Each of the following items equals 1 serving.

Breads
  Bagel, small, ½
  Dinner roll, 1
  Dried bread crumbs, 3 tablespoons
  English muffin, small, ½
  Tortilla (6 inch), 1
  Whole wheat, rye, or pumpernickel, 1 slice
Cereals
  Bran flakes, ½ cup
  Cornmeal (dry), 2 tablespoons
  Flour, 2½ tablespoons
  Grits (cooked), ½ cup
  Pasta (cooked), ½ cup
  Porridge (cooked cereal), ½ cup
  Puffed cereal (unsweetened), 1 cup
  Rice or barley (cooked), ½ cup
  Unpuffed, unsweetened cereal, ¾ cup
  Wheat germ, ¼ cup
Crackers
  Arrowroot, 3
  Graham (2½-inch squares), 2

Matzo (4 by 6 inches), ½

Rye wafers (2 by 3½ inches), 3

Saltine, 6

Starchy vegetables

Corn, kernels, ⅓ cup

Corn on cob, 1 small cob

Parsnips, ⅔ cup

Potato, mashed, ½ cup

Potato, white, 1 small

Squash (winter, acorn, or butternut), ½ cup

Yam or sweet potato, ¼ cup

Prepared foods

Each of the following items equals 2 servings.

Biscuit, 2-inch diameter (omit 1 fat exchange), 1

Corn bread, 2 by 2 by 1 inch (omit 1 fat exchange), 1

French fries, 2 to 3 inches long (omit 1 fat exchange), 8

Muffin, small (omit 1 fat exchange), 1

Pancake, 5 by ½ inch (omit 1 fat exchange), 1

Waffle, 5 by ½ inch (omit 1 fat exchange), 1

The following item equals 3 servings

Potato or corn chips, 15

List 4: Legumes

According to the dictionary, a legume is a plant that produces a pod that splits on both sides. Of the common human foods, beans, peas, lentils, and peanuts are legumes. The legume category also includes alfalfa, clover, acacia, and indigo. The fossil record indicates that legumes are among the oldest cultivated plants; prehistoric peoples domesticated and cultivated certain legumes for food. Today, legumes are a mainstay in most diets of the world. Legumes are second only to grains in supplying calories and protein to the human population. Compared to grains, they supply about the same number of total calories, but usually provide two to four times as much protein. Legumes are often called "the poor people's meat"; they might be better known as "the healthy people's meat." Although lacking some key amino acids, legumes can be combined with grains to form what is known as a complete protein.

Legumes are fantastic foods. They are rich in important nutrients and health-promoting compounds. Legumes help improve liver function and lower cholesterol levels. They are extremely effective in improving blood sugar control. One study conducted over a four-year period involved over 175 elderly men and women between the ages of 64 and 87. Their habitual intake of legumes was inversely related to the incidence of glucose intolerance and diabetes.[12] In other words, the higher the intake of legumes, the greater the protection against blood sugar abnormalities. Since obesity and diabetes have been linked to blood sugar volatility (insulin insensitivity), legumes are extremely important in weight-loss plans and in the dietary management of diabetes.

Legumes

In this list, ½ cup of each item, cooked or sprouted, equals 1 serving.

Black-eyed peas

Chickpeas

Garbanzo beans

Kidney beans

Lentils

Lima beans

Pinto beans

Split peas

Other dried beans and peas

The following item, in a quantity of ½ cup, equals 2 servings.

Soybeans, including tofu

List 5: Fats and Oils

Saturated fats are known to have a negative effect on glucose control. They are linked to both diabetes and hypoglycemia. Typical saturated fats are animal fats and are solid at room temperature. In contrast, vegetable fats are liquid at room temperature and are referred to as unsaturated fats or oils. The human body requires certain fats; they are essential. Specifically, the human body requires the fatty acids linoleic acid and linolenic acid. These fatty acids function as components of nerve cells, cellular membranes, and hormone-like substances known as prostaglandins. (Prostaglandins stimulate contraction of smooth muscle, lower blood pressure, regulate body temperature and blood clotting, and help control inflammation.) Increased consumption of essential fatty acids has been shown to lower the cholesterol level and improve many symptoms of diabetes.

Although essential fatty acids are critical to human health, too much fat in the diet, especially saturated fat, is linked to numerous cancers, heart disease, and stroke. Most nutrition experts strongly recommend that total daily fat intake be kept below 30% of total daily calories. In addition, they recommend that people eat at least twice as much unsaturated fat as saturated fat. This recommendation is easy to follow. Simply reduce the amount of animal products in the diet; increase the amount of nuts and seeds; and use natural polyunsaturated oils—such as canola, safflower, soy, and flaxseed—as salad dressings.

Most commercially available salad dressings, as well as those in restaurants, are full of the wrong type of oil. Try the recipe for Basil Dressing, which appears later in this chapter. It includes polyunsaturated and therapeutic vegetable oils in a delicious combination.

In addition to saturated fats, avoid margarine. During the manufacture of margarine and shortening, vegetable oils are hydrogenated. This means that a hydrogen molecule is added to the natural unsaturated fatty-acid molecule of a vegetable oil to make it saturated. Hydrogenation changes the liquid vegetable oil to a solid or semisolid.

Many researchers and nutritionists have been concerned about the health effects of margarine since it was introduced. Although many Americans assume they are doing their body good by consuming margarine instead of butter, they are actually doing harm. Margarine and other hydrogenated vegetable oils not only raise LDL cholesterol; they lower the protective HDL cholesterol level, interfere with essential fatty acid metabolism, and are suspected of causing certain cancers.[13] If you desire a butterlike spread, use a canola-oil product that is nonhydrogenated.

Perhaps the best way of increasing the intake of essential fatty acids is increasing the consumption of nuts and seeds. Nuts and seeds are especially good sources of essential fatty acids, vitamin E, protein, minerals, fiber, and other health-promoting substances.

Because of the high oil content of nuts and seeds, you might suspect that their frequent consumption would increase obesity. But a large population study of 26,473 Americans revealed that those who consumed the most nuts were less obese. This statistic is quite interesting. A possible explanation is that the nuts produced satiety, a feeling of appetite satisfaction. This study also demonstrated that high nut consumption was associated with fewer heart attacks (both fatal and nonfatal).[14]

The results of a recent study designed to investigate the protective effects of walnuts against heart disease were published in the prestigious *New England Journal of Medicine.* The researchers found that walnut consumption lowered total cholesterol 12.4%, reduced LDL cholesterol 16.3%, and decreased triglyceride levels 8.3% in men with normal blood lipid levels.[15] Presumably, other nuts exert similar effects on blood lipids. The beneficial effects are thought to be due to the oils in nuts.

Many physicians use a preparation of flaxseed, in combination with evening primrose and black-currant oil, for medicinal purposes. Although this combination can be effective, patients may realize better results by consuming whole nuts and seeds. Compared to nut oil in medicinal preparations, the oil in fresh nuts and seeds is less likely to be rancid, and the whole nut or seed contains many helpful substances in addition to the oil.

In general, nuts and seeds, due to their high oil content, are best purchased and stored in their shells. The shell is a natural protector against light and air, which promote damage by free radicals. Make sure the shells are free from splits, cracks, stains, holes, or other surface imperfections. Do not eat or use moldy nuts or seeds; eating them may not be safe. Also avoid limp, rubbery, dark, or shriveled nutmeats. Store nuts and seeds, in their shells, in a cool, dry environment. If unavailable in their shells, store nutmeats and shelled seeds in airtight containers in the refrigerator or freezer. Crushed and slivered nuts and nut pieces are the nut products that are most often rancid. Prepare your own nutmeats from whole nuts.

Try to eat at least 2 servings of nuts per day. Note that, in the Healthy Exchange System, cream is in the fats and oils list.

Fats and Oils

Each of the following items equals 1 serving.

Mono-unsaturated
Olive oil, 1 teaspoon
Olives, 5 small
Polyunsaturated
Almonds, 10 whole
Avocado (4-inch diameter), 1/8 fruit
Peanuts
    Spanish, 20 whole
    Virginia, 10 whole
Pecans, 2 large
Seeds, 1 tablespoon
    Flax
    Pumpkin
    Sesame
    Sunflower
Vegetable oil, 1 teaspoon
    Canola
    Corn
    Flax
    Safflower
    Soy
    Sunflower
Walnuts, 6 small
Saturated (use sparingly)
Bacon, 1 slice
Butter, 1 teaspoon
Cream, heavy, 1 tablespoon
Cream, light or sour, 2 tablespoons
Cream cheese, 1 tablespoon
Mayonnaise, 1 teaspoon
Salad dressing, 2 teaspoons

List 6: Milk

Is milk for everybody? Definitely not. Many people are allergic to milk or lack the enzymes necessary to digest it. The drinking of cow's milk is a relatively new dietary practice for humans. This may be the reason so many people have difficulty with milk. Evidence has shown that an infant's early exposure to cow's milk is a trigger to developing type I diabetes.[16] Several studies have shown that the consumption of milk is directly related to the development of type I diabetes. Other studies have shown that children under one year of age should not drink cow's milk; older children and adults should drink no more than 2 servings per day. Choose nonfat products.

Another reason to avoid cow's milk is that a milk protein known as casein appears to promote atherosclerosis.[17] Many meal-replacement formulas, including Ultra Slim Fast, contain casein. Casein is also used in glues, molded plastics, and paints. A good alternative to cow's milk and casein-containing formulas is soy milk or soy-based formulas. Unlike casein, soy protein actually lowers cholesterol.[18]

Milk

In each of the following items one cup equals 1 serving.

Nonfat milk or yogurt

Nonfat soy milk

Lowfat yogurt (omit 1 fat exchange)

2% milk (omit 1 fat exchange)

Whole milk (omit 2 fat exchanges)

Yogurt (omit 2 fat exchanges)

List 7: Meats, Fish, Cheese, and Eggs

When choosing from this list, choose primarily from the lowfat group and remove the skin of poultry. This will keep the amount of saturated fat low. List 7 provides high concentrations of certain nutrients difficult to get in an entirely vegetarian diet. It provides the full range of amino acids, vitamin B12, and iron. The most important recommendation may be to use these foods in small amounts. Think of them as condiments in the diet rather than mainstays.

Diabetics, children, and all health-minded individuals should not eat smoked or cured meat. Evidence suggests that eating smoked or cured meat can lead to diabetes. Smoked or cured meat, like pickled vegetables, is rich in compounds that can lead to the formation of nitrosamines. Dietary nitrosamines can damage the beta cells of the pancreas. In one study, when 339 children with type I diabetes were compared to 528 nondiabetic children, researchers found that the diabetic children had a high frequency of nitrosamine consumption.[19] A compound similar to a nitrosamine, streptozotocin, is used to cause diabetes in animals used in experiments. (Streptozotocin destroys the insulin-producing beta cells of the pancreas.)

A possible exception to the recommendation of reducing the intake of animal foods is cold-water fish such as salmon, mackerel, and herring. These fish contain oils known as omega-3 fatty acids. Hundreds of studies have shown that these beneficial oils lower cholesterol and triglyceride levels. Many of these studies included diabetics. The omega-3 fatty acids are not only being recommended to treat or prevent high cholesterol levels; they are also being recommended to treat or prevent high blood pressure and other cardiovascular diseases; cancer; autoimmune diseases, such as multiple sclerosis and rheumatoid arthritis; allergies and inflammation; eczema; psoriasis; and many others.[20] The majority of studies of omega-3 fatty acids have utilized fish oils (eicosapentaenoic acid [EPA] and docosahexaenoic acid [DHA]). Vegans may be able to derive benefits similar to these offered by fish oils by consuming flaxseed oil. It contains linolenic acid, an omega-3 oil that the body can convert to EPA. Linolenic acid exerts many of the same effects as EPA as well as several others.

A substantial body of evidence documents the relationship between increasing the intake of fish oils and lowering blood cholesterol. The question remains, however: Should fish oils be taken as a supplement, or should the dietary intake of fish be increased? In an effort to resolve this question, a recent study of 25 men with high cholesterol levels compared, over a five-week period, the effects of eating an equivalent amount of fish oil from whole fish versus those of consuming a fish-oil supplement.[21] Although total cholesterol levels were unchanged in both groups, both fish and fish-oil supplements lowered triglycerides and raised HDL cholesterol.

However, dietary fish produced some benefits that fish-oil supplements did not. In this study dietary fish oil was more effective than the fish-oil supplement in reducing platelet "stickiness." When platelets are sticky and adhere to each other, they can form a clot. This clot can get stuck in small arteries and produce a heart attack or stroke. These findings suggest that, though both fish consumption and fish-oil supplements produce desirable effects on lipids and lipoproteins, fish consumption is more effective in improving several other factors involved in cardiovascular disease.

Meats, Fish, Cheese, and Eggs

Low fat (less than 15% fat)

Each of the following items equals 1 serving.

Beef, 1 ounce

Baby, chipped, chuck

Round (bottom, top), rump (all cuts), steak (flank, plate), spareribs, tenderloin plate ribs, tripe

Cottage cheese, low fat, ¼ cup

Fish, 1 ounce

Lamb, 1 ounce

   Leg, loin (roast and chops), rib, shank, sirloin, shoulder

Poultry, chicken or turkey without skin, 1 ounce

Veal, 1 ounce

   Cutlet, leg, loin, rib, shank, shoulder

Medium fat (for each omit ½ fat exchange):

Beef, 1 ounce

   Canned corned, ground (15% fat), rib eye, round (ground commercial)

Cheese, 1 ounce

   Farmer, Mozzarella, Parmesan, ricotta

Eggs, 1

Organ meats, 1 ounce

Peanut butter, 2 tablespoons

Pork, 1 ounce

   Boiled, Boston butt, Canadian bacon, loin (all tenderloin), picnic

High fat (for each exchange omit 1 fat exchange):

Beef, 1 ounce

   Brisket, corned, ground (more than 20% fat), hamburger (less than 20% fat), roasts (rib), steaks (club and rib)

Cheese, cheddar, 1 ounce

Duck or goose, 1 ounce

Lamb breast, 1 ounce

Pork, 1 ounce

   Country-style ham, deviled ham, ground, loin, spareribs

Menu Planning

The Healthy Exchange System was created to ensure that you are consuming a diet that is providing adequate nutrients in their proper ratio. To construct a daily menu, you must first have determined your caloric needs and learned the number of servings required from each healthy exchange list.

Breakfast

Breakfast is an absolute must. Healthful breakfast choices include whole grain cereals, muffins, and breads, along with fresh fruit or fresh fruit juice. Hot or cold cereal, preferably from whole grains, may be the best choice for breakfast. The complex carbohydrates in the grains provide sustained energy, and evidence shows that eating whole grains at breakfast can lower cholesterol. An evaluation of data from the National Health and Nutrition Examination Survey II (a national survey of the nutrition and health practices of Americans) disclosed that blood cholesterol levels are lowest among adults eating whole-grain cereal for breakfast.[22] Those individuals who consumed other breakfast foods had higher blood cholesterol levels than those who ate whole grains. Levels were highest among those who skipped breakfast.

Thanks to an explosion of marketing information, most Americans are aware of the cholesterol-lowering effects of oats. Since 1963, there have been over 20 major clinical studies examining the effect of oat bran on cholesterol levels.[23] Various oat preparations containing either oat bran or oatmeal have been studied, including cereals, muffins, breads, and entrées. The overwhelming majority of the studies demonstrated a very favorable effect on cholesterol levels. In individuals with high cholesterol levels (above 220 milligrams per deciliter), the consumption of the equivalent of 3 grams of water-soluble oat fiber lowered total cholesterol by 8% to 23%. One bowl of ready-to-eat oat bran cereal provides approximately 3 grams of fiber. Although the fiber content of oatmeal (7%) is less than that of oat bran (15% to 26%), studies have determined that the polyunsaturated fatty acids from the oatmeal contribute as much to the cholesterol-lowering effects of oats as the fiber content. Although oat bran has a higher fiber content, oatmeal is higher in polyunsaturated fatty acids. This makes oat bran and oatmeal equally effective. Here are a couple of breakfast suggestions.

Happy Apple Breakfast

Makes 2 servings

1½	cups rolled oats*
2½	cups water
1	sliced medium green *or* golden apple
½	teaspoon cinnamon
¼	cup currants, raisins, *or* chopped dates (*optional*)
¼	cup pumpkin seeds, fresh *or* roasted (*optional*)
	Honey, to taste (*optional*)

In a medium saucepan, combine oats and water. Bring mixture to a boil, then simmer for 10 minutes. Cover and remove from heat. Let stand 5 more minutes. While oats stand, combine remaining ingredients in a medium bowl. Serve oat mixture, using apple mixture as a topping.

Dietary Servings Per Recipe Serving
Fruits: ½
Grains and starches: 2

Nutrition Information Per Recipe Serving
Calories: 184
Carbohydrate: 73%

Protein: 15%
Fat: 12%
Fiber: 2 grams
Calcium: 37 milligrams

*Instead of some or all of the rolled oats, other rolled grains—such as wheat, barley, rye, or triticale—can be used in various combinations. All these grains have the same cooking characteristics. This oatmeal dish need not be served with milk, and the nutrition information for the recipe does not include milk.

Bran Muffins

Makes 12 servings (1 muffin per serving)

1¼	cups whole-wheat flour
1	cup wheat bran*
1	teaspoon baking soda
1	teaspoon cinnamon
⅛	cup canola oil
⅓ to ½	cup honey
1	cup nonfat milk
½	teaspoon vanilla
	Canola oil, to grease tin

Preheat oven to 400 degrees F. In a medium bowl, combine all the dry ingredients. In a large bowl, mix all the liquid ingredients. Add dry ingredients to liquid ingredients; mix until ingredients are just combined. While mixture stands, oil one muffin tin; sprinkle each cup with flour. Spoon batter into each cup until it is half full. Bake for 25 minutes.

Dietary Servings Per Recipe Serving
Fruits: ½
Grains and starches: 1

ᐳ

Fats: ⅓
Milk: ¹⁄₁₂

Nutrition Information Per Recipe Serving
Calories: 114
Carbohydrate: 70%
Protein: 10%
Fat: 20%
Fiber: 3 grams
Calcium: 34 milligrams
*Oat bran can be substituted for wheat bran.

Lunch

Lunch is a great time to enjoy a healthful bowl of soup, a large salad, and some whole-grain bread. For people with diabetes or hypoglycemia, bean soups and other legume dishes are especially good lunch selections, because these dishes can improve blood sugar regulation. Legumes are filling, yet low in calories.

Many of the recipes that appear in the remainder of this chapter call for Lite Salt or a salt substitute as an ingredient. Lite Salt is a product that includes more potassium chloride than sodium chloride. (It contains 190 milligrams of sodium chloride per gram.) Lite Salt is manufactured by Morton International, Incorporated, of Chicago, and it is available in most full-service supermarkets. A similar product is Nu-Salt, from the Cumberland Packing Corporation of New York. The term *salt substitute* refers to a number of commercially available herbal mixtures (such as Spike, a product of Modern Seasoning of Milwaukee) as well as natural seasoning products (such as toasted seaweed). These may be available in supermarkets, though you will probably have better luck finding them in health food stores.

Lentil Soup

Makes 6 servings

1	tablespoon olive oil
2	large onions, finely diced
4	cloves garlic, minced
2	green peppers, finely diced
10	cups vegetable stock, homemade or store-bought
2	carrots, thinly sliced
1½	cups lentils, rinsed, with imperfect lentils removed
⅓	teaspoon thyme
	Freshly ground black pepper, to taste
½	teaspoon Lite Salt *or* salt substitute
1	can (28 ounces) plum tomatoes, with juice, finely chopped
1	pound loose fresh spinach, stems removed, finely chopped *or* 1 package (10 ounces) frozen chopped spinach, thawed

In a large stockpot over medium heat, heat oil. Add onions, garlic, and green peppers; sauté for 10 minutes. Add vegetable stock, carrots, lentils, and thyme. Bring stock to a boil. Reduce heat. Simmer, stirring occasionally, until lentils are tender (about 45 minutes). Add spinach; cook until spinach has wilted and become tender (about 5 minutes). Season with pepper and Lite Salt.

Dietary Servings Per Recipe Serving
Vegetables: 1
Legumes: 1
Fats: ½

Nutrition Information Per Recipe Serving
Calories: 182
Carbohydrate: 54%
Protein: 16%
Fat: 30%
Fiber: 2 grams
Calcium: 137 milligrams

Served with bread, this soup provides excellent protein.

Dark Peasant Bread

Makes 8 servings (one loaf)

1½	cups very warm water
1½	tablespoons dry yeast
¼	cup molasses
4–4½	cups whole-wheat flour
1	cup rye flour
2	teaspoons caraway seed
¼	cup carob powder, sifted
	Canola oil, for greasing

In a large bowl, combine the water, yeast, and molasses. Let stand until bubbly (about 10 minutes). Beat in 2 cups of the whole-wheat flour. With a towel, cover bowl loosely. Place bowl in warm area until the mixture has doubled in bulk (about 20 minutes). Stir in rye flour, caraway seed, and carob powder. Then add, 1 cup at a time, enough of the remaining whole-wheat flour to make a soft dough that can be kneaded. Knead well, about 5 minutes. Clean and oil the bowl. Place dough in bowl and cover loosely with a towel. Let dough rise until doubled (30 to 40 minutes). Oil one standard-sized loaf pan. Punch down dough and knead.

Shape dough into loaf and place in pan. Let dough rise again, until doubled in bulk. While dough rises, preheat oven to 350 degrees F. Bake loaf for 40 to 45 minutes.

Dietary Servings Per Recipe Serving
Grains and starches: 3

Nutrition Information Per Recipe Serving
Calories: 210
Carbohydrate: 85%
Protein: 12%
Fat: 3%
Fiber: 7 grams
Calcium: 49 milligrams

This is an interesting bread that is certainly worth a try, especially if you like rye.

Insalata Mista Salad

Makes 4 servings

1	head lettuce
1	fennel bulb
½	small cucumber, sliced
6	radishes, trimmed and sliced
1	celery heart, chopped
1	small green pepper, cored, seeded, and sliced
4	scallions, thinly sliced
2	ripe, firm tomatoes
	Lite Salt *or* salt substitute, to taste
2	tablespoons olive oil
2	teaspoons cider vinegar *or* lemon juice

Pull off and discard bruised or blemished lettuce leaves. Wash and dry remaining leaves; tear into bite-sized pieces and place in a large salad bowl. Trim off the stalks, base, and coarse outer leaves from fennel; cut downward into thin slices, then cut into strips. Add fennel to the salad bowl, along with cucumber, radishes, celery, pepper, and scallions. Cut tomatoes into eighths; add to the bowl. When ready to serve, sprinkle salad with Lite Salt. Add olive oil and cider vinegar; toss lightly. Serve immediately.

Dietary Servings Per Recipe Serving
Vegetables: ¾
Fats: ½

Nutrition Information Per Recipe Serving
Calories: 70
Carbohydrate: 52%
Protein: 19%
Fat: 30%
Fiber: 5 grams
Calcium: 50 milligrams

This salad is low in calories, but high in nutrition.

Snacks

The best snacks to help control blood sugar levels are nuts, seeds, and fresh fruits and vegetables. Choose foods with a low glycemic index (see Chapter 5).

Dinner

For dinner, the healthiest meals contain a fresh vegetable salad, a cooked vegetable side dish or a bowl of soup, whole grains, and legumes. The whole grains may be in bread, pasta, pizza, or as a side dish or part of an entrée. The legumes can be in a soup, salad, or entrée.

Although a diet rich in whole grains, vegetables, and legumes provides optimal levels of protein, some people like to eat meat. The important thing is not to overconsume animal products. Limit your intake to no more than 4 to 6 ounces per day and select fish, skinless poultry, and lean cuts rather than fat-ladened choices.

Basil Dressing

Makes 6 servings (2 tablespoons per serving)

¼   cup vegetable oil
3   tablespoons fresh lemon juice
¼   cup water
2   tablespoons minced fresh basil *or* 1½ teaspoons dried basil
1   teaspoon finely chopped garlic
     Black pepper, to taste

Combine all ingredients in a blender or food processor. Blend thoroughly.

Orange and Fennel Salad

Makes 4 servings

2   large fennel bulbs *or* 4 small fennel bulbs
4   oranges
1   medium lemon
1   tablespoon olive oil
     Lite Salt *or* salt substitute, to taste
     Freshly ground black pepper, to taste
8   black olives *(optional)*

Wash, trim, and cut fennel lengthwise, into thick wedges. Cut the tops and bottoms off oranges. To peel, hold each one over a serving dish and use a small sharp or serrated knife to cut away the peel and white pith. Slice across the segments and arrange orange pieces and fennel in a shallow serving dish. Cut off peel and pith from half the lemon; chop the flesh. Sprinkle chopped lemon over orange and fennel. Pour olive oil over mixture in bowl; add lemon juice to taste, from the remaining lemon half. Season with Lite Salt and pepper. Toss well. Cover and chill until required. Just before serving, decorate salad with black olives if desired.

Dietary Servings Per Recipe Serving
Vegetables: 1
Fruits: 1
Fats: 1

Nutrition Information Per Recipe Serving
Calories: 170
Carbohydrate: 58%
Protein: 12%
Fat: 30%
Fiber: 3.5 grams
Calcium: 100 milligrams

The combination of the flavonoids in the orange and the coumarins in the fennel offers healing features.

Polenta Puttanesca

Makes 4 servings

Polenta

4   cups water
1¼   cups cornmeal
⅓   teaspoon Lite Salt *or* salt substitute

Sauce

1	tablespoon olive oil
7 or more	cloves garlic, peeled and chopped
¼	teaspoon dried red pepper flakes
2	large green peppers, cut into strips
2	pounds tomatoes, chopped and drained
2	tablespoons tomato paste
6	black olives, halved
2	teaspoons capers
¼	teaspoon Lite Salt *or* salt substitute
	Freshly ground black pepper, to taste
⅓	cup grated soy cheese.

In a large saucepan, bring the water to a boil. Drizzle in the cornmeal slowly, whisking continuously with a wire whisk. Add Lite Salt; reduce heat to low. Continue to whisk as mixture thickens. Stir until polenta pulls away from the sides of the pan (5 to 7 minutes). Top each serving of polenta with sauce, then top sauce with soy cheese. Serve immediately.

Sauce   In a large skillet, heat oil over medium heat. Add garlic and red pepper flakes. Cook for 3 minutes. Add green peppers; sauté 10 minutes. Add tomatoes, tomato paste, olives, capers, Lite Salt, and pepper. Cook until peppers are tender and sauce thickens (about 30 minutes).

Dietary Servings Per Recipe Serving
Vegetables: 1½
Grains and starches: 2
Fats: 1
Milk: ¹/₈

Nutrition Information Per Recipe Serving
Calories: 254
Carbohydrate: 61%

Protein: 9%
Fat: 30%
Fiber: 3 grams
Calcium: 192 milligrams

Instead of adding tomatoes and tomato paste, you can add 16 ounces of an all-natural spaghetti sauce. This dish is one of my favorites. It is a great way to get your daily quota of garlic.

Chapter Summary

A diet high in complex carbohydrates and dietary fiber and low in fat is clearly the diet of choice in the treatment of diabetes and hypoglycemia. The Healthy Exchange System presented in this chapter allows for the construction of such a diet. It is important to recognize that, whenever a type I diabetic changes his or her diet, insulin dosage or schedule may have to be altered.

7

Essential Substances in Blood Sugar Control

The treatment of diabetes and hypoglycemia requires nutritional supplementation. Diabetics and hypoglycemics have such an increased need for many nutrients that dietary supplementation is the only practical solution.[1] Supplying these people with additional key nutrients has been shown to improve blood sugar control as well as help prevent or improve many of the major complications of their conditions.

A good way to start a supplementation program is to begin taking a high-quality multiple vitamin and mineral formula—one that provides adequate levels of the key nutrients people with diabetes or hypoglycemia require. (Many supplement manufacturers provide specific formulas to support an individual with diabetes or hypoglycemia.) This chapter will outline what those nutrition requirements are.

Although nutritional supplementation will go a long way in helping prevent many of the major complications of diabetes and hypoglycemia, keep in mind the fact that supplements should be used only as a part of a comprehensive treatment approach. Diet, not supplements, should be the primary focus.

Chromium

The importance of chromium to human nutrition was not discovered until 1957. Chromium is vital to blood sugar control. Chromium works closely with insulin in facilitating the uptake of glucose into cells. Without chromium, the action of insulin is blocked and the level of glucose rises.

In some clinical studies of diabetics, supplementing the diet with chromium has been shown to decrease fasting glucose levels, improve glucose tolerance, lower insulin levels, and decrease total cholesterol and triglyceride levels while increasing the level of HDL cholesterol.[2] Although other studies have not shown chromium to exert much effect in improving glucose tolerance in diabetes, there is no argument that chromium is an important mineral in blood sugar metabolism.

Chromium plays an important role in hypoglycemia as well. In one study, eight female patients with hypoglycemia received 200 micrograms of chromium per day for three months. The women's symptoms of hypoglycemia were alleviated.[3] In addition, glucose tolerance test results improved and the number of insulin receptors on red blood cells increased.

In addition, research has shown that reversing a chromium deficiency by supplementing the diet with chromium can lower body weight and increase lean body mass. All the effects of chromium appear to be due to increased insulin sensitivity. A chromium deficiency may be an underlying factor in the cases of the many Americans who have diabetes, hypoglycemia, and are obese. There is evidence that marginal chromium deficiency is quite common in the United States.

Although there is no recommended dietary allowance (RDA) for chromium, it appears that humans need at least 200 micrograms each day. Chromium in the body can be depleted by eating refined sugars, white-flour products and by lack of exercise. In addition to the regular consumption of chromium-rich foods, the diabetic and hypoglycemic should supplement the diet with 200 to 400 micrograms of chromium each day. Chromium polynicotinate, chromium picolinate, and chromium-enriched yeast are suitable forms of dietary supplements.

Vitamin C

Vitamin C is perhaps the most publicized vitamin. The primary function of vitamin C is in the manufacture of collagen, the main protein substance of the human body. Since collagen is such an important protein in the structures that hold the body together (connective tissue, cartilage, tendons, and so on), vitamin C is vital for wound repair, healthy gums, and the prevention of easy bruising. In scurvy, or severe vitamin C deficiency, the classic symptoms are bleeding gums, poor wound healing, and extensive bruising. Susceptibility to infection, hysteria, and depression are also hallmarks. In addition to its role in collagen metabolism, vitamin C is critical to immune function, the manufacture of certain hormones and transmitting substances in nerves, and the absorption and utilization of other nutritional substances.

The debate over how much vitamin C humans need is ongoing. At one end of the spectrum, two-time Nobel Prize winner Linus Pauling and his followers recommend an intake of 2 to 9 grams per day during periods of health and even higher doses during times of stress or illness. At the other end of the spectrum, the RDA of vitamin C for adults is 60 milligrams. For diabetics, Pauling's recommendations appear to be more appropriate.

Since insulin facilitates the transport of vitamin C into cells, many diabetics do not have enough vitamin C inside the cells of their bodies.[4] Therefore, these people have a vitamin C deficiency, although they seem to take an adequate dietary amount. The fact is, diabetics need more vitamin C than healthy nondiabetics. A chronic, latent vitamin C deficiency can lead to a number of problems for the diabetic. These include an increased tendency to bleed (increased capillary permeability), poor wound healing, an elevated cholesterol level, and a depressed immune system. Furthermore, research has shown that vitamin C at high doses (1 to 2 grams per day) reduces the accumulation of sorbitol within cells and inhibits the glycosylation of proteins.[5] As Chapter 2 discussed, sorbitol accumulation and glycosylation of proteins are linked to many complications of diabetes, especially eye and nerve diseases.

Although vitamin C supplementation will be necessary to reach an intake of at least 2 grams per day, do not rely exclusively on supplements to meet all your vitamin C requirements. Vitamin C–rich foods are rich in compounds, such as flavonoids and carotenes, that work to enhance the effects of vitamin C as well as exert favorable effects of their own.

Most people think of citrus fruits as the best source of vitamin C. Vegetables also contain high levels—especially broccoli, peppers, potatoes, and Brussels sprouts. Vitamin C is destroyed by exposure to air. So, eat fresh produce as soon as possible. Although a salad from a salad bar is a healthier choice than a processed meal, the vitamin C content of the fruits and vegetables is only a fraction of what it would be if the salad was fresh. For example, freshly sliced cucumbers, if left standing, lose 41% to 49% of their vitamin C content within the first three hours. A sliced cantaloupe, if left uncovered in the refrigerator, loses 35% of the vitamin C content in less than 24 hours.

Table 7.1   Vitamin C Content of Selected Foods, in Milligrams, per 3½-oz (100-g) Serving

Acerola	1,300	Liver, calf	36
Peppers, red chili	369	Turnips	36
Guavas	242	Mangoes	35
Peppers, red sweet	190	Asparagus	33
Kale leaves	186	Cantaloupe	33
Parsley	172	Swiss chard	32
Collard leaves	152	Green onions	32
Turnip greens	139	Liver, beef	31
Peppers, green sweet	128	Okra	31
Broccoli	113	Tangerines	31
Brussels sprouts	102	New Zealand spinach	30
Mustard greens	97	Oysters	30
Watercress	79	Lima beans, young	29
Cauliflower	78	Black-eyed peas	29
Persimmons	66	Soybeans	29
Cabbage, red	61	Green peas	27
Strawberries	59	Radishes	26
Papayas	56	Raspberries	25
Spinach	51	Chinese cabbage	25
Oranges and juice	50	Yellow summer squash	25
Cabbage	47	Loganberries	24
Lemon juice	46	Honeydew melon	23
Grapefruit and juice	38	Tomatoes	23
Elderberries	36	Liver, pork	23

SOURCE: "Nutritive Value of American Foods in Common Units," U.S.D.A. Agriculture Handbook No. 456.

Table 7.1 cites the vitamin C content of selected foods.

Niacin and Niacinamide

Enzymes containing niacin (vitamin B3) play an important role in energy production; fat, cholesterol, and carbohydrate metabolism; and the manufacture of many body compounds, including sex and adrenal hormones. Niacin, like chromium, facilitates the uptake of glucose, making it a key nutrient in the treatment of hypoglycemia and diabetes.[6]

Supplementing the diet of diabetics with niacin in the form of niacinamide can have many favorable effects. Foremost is the possible prevention of diabetes.[7] Niacinamide, also called nicotinamide, has been shown to prevent the development of diabetes in experimental animals. This observation led to several pilot clinical studies. The results of these studies suggested that niacinamide can prevent type I diabetes from developing. Or, if given soon enough at the onset of diabetes, it can help restore beta cells or at least slow down their destruction. Some newly diagnosed type I diabetics have experienced complete resolution of their diabetes after niacinamide supplementation.[8] In 1992, researchers launched a study involving 18 European countries, Israel, and Canada to follow up these preliminary findings. Other clinical trials are also in progress.

When used as a supplement in the treatment of diabetes or hyperglycemia, the dose of nicotinamide is based on body weight, roughly 25 milligrams per 2 pounds. The studies in children used 100 to 200 milligrams per day. When niacin therapy is being used to reduce a high cholesterol level, it is important to use inositol hexaniacinate rather than regular niacin. Of the two, inositol hexaniacinate is easier to tolerate, and it has not been shown to impair glucose tolerance.

Biotin

Biotin is a B vitamin that functions in the manufacture and utilization of carbohydrates, fats, and amino acids. Without biotin, metabolism is severely impaired. Biotin is manufactured in the intestines by bacteria. A vegetarian diet has been shown to alter the intestinal bacterial flora in such a manner as to enhance the synthesis and promote the absorption of biotin.

Biotin supplementation can enhance insulin sensitivity and increase the activity of the enzyme glucokinase. Glucokinase is the enzyme responsible for the first step in the utilization of glucose by the liver. In diabetics, glucokinase concentrations are very low. Evidently, supplementing the diet with high doses of biotin improves glucokinase activity and glucose metabolism in diabetics. In one study, 16 milligrams of biotin per day resulted in a significant lowering of fasting blood sugar levels and improvements in blood glucose control in type I diabetics.[9] In a study of type II diabetics, similar effects were noted with 9 milligrams of biotin per day.[10]

If high-dose biotin is used in type I diabetics, insulin requirements must be adjusted. Supervision by a physician is required.

Vitamin B6

Pyridoxine, one form of vitamin B6, is extremely important in the formation of body proteins and structural compounds, chemical transmitters in the nervous system, red blood cells, and hormonelike compounds known as prostaglandins. Vitamin B6 is also critical in maintaining hormone balance and proper immune function.

Deficiency of vitamin B6 is characterized by depression, convulsions (especially in children), glucose intolerance, and impaired nerve function. Although extreme deficiency of vitamin B6 is believed to be quite rare, numerous clinical studies have demonstrated that a number of health conditions respond to B6 supplementation. These conditions include asthma, premenstrual syndrome (PMS), carpal tunnel syndrome, depression, morning sickness, and kidney stones. It is of interest that the increased rate of these disorders since the 1950s parallels the increased levels of substances in the food supply that are antagonistic to vitamin B6. These antagonists to vitamin B6 include the hydrazine dyes (FD&C yellow #5), certain drugs (isoniazid, hydralazine, dopamine, and penicillamine), oral contraceptives, alcohol, and excessive protein. The intake of the dye yellow #5 is often consumed in greater quantities than the RDA for vitamin B6, or 2.0 milligrams for males and 1.6 milligrams for females. (The per capita intake of yellow #5 is 15 grams per day.)

Vitamin B6 supplementation appears to offer significant protection against the development of diabetic neuropathy, in that diabetics with neuropathy have been shown to be deficient in vitamin B6 and benefit from supplementation.[11] The neuropathy of a vitamin B6 deficiency is indistinguishable from a diabetic neuropathy. Individuals with long-standing diabetes or who are developing signs of peripheral nerve abnormalities should definitely supplement their diets with vitamin B6. The standard daily dose for this application is 150 milligrams.

Vitamin B6 may also prove to be important in preventing other diabetic complications, because it inhibits glycosylation of proteins.[12] Vitamin B6 supplementation is a safe treatment for gestational diabetes (diabetes caused by pregnancy). In one study, 14 women with gestational diabetes took 100 mg of vitamin B6 for two weeks. The result was elimination of the diabetes in 12 of the 14 women.[13]

Vitamin B12

Vitamin B12—in particular, cobalamin, a component of the vitamin—was isolated from a liver extract in 1948 and identified as the nutritional factor which prevented pernicious anemia. Because of its cobalt content, vitamin B12 is a bright red crystalline compound. The vitamin works with folic acid in many body processes, including the synthesis of DNA. Since vitamin B12 works to reactivate folic acid, a deficiency of B12 results in a folic acid deficiency if folic acid levels are marginal.

A vitamin B12 deficiency is characterized by numbness of the feet, "pins-and-needles" sensations, or a burning feeling. In the elderly, a vitamin B12 deficiency can cause impaired mental function that mimics Alzheimer's disease. Vitamin B12 deficiency is thought to be quite common in the elderly. In addition to depression or mental confusion, its symptoms can be anemia; a smooth, beefy red tongue; and diarrhea.

Vitamin B12 is necessary in only very small quantities. The RDA is 2 micrograms. Vitamin B12 is found in significant quantities only in foods derived from animals. The richest sources are liver and kidney, followed by eggs, fish, cheese, and meat. Strict vegetarians (vegans) are often told that fermented foods such as tempeh are excellent sources of vitamin B12. However, in addition to tremendous variation of B12 content in fermented foods, there is some evidence that the form of B12 in these foods is not exactly the form that meets body requirements. Although the vitamin B12 content of certain cooked sea vegetables is in the same range as that of beef, researchers do not know if the body can use the form of B12 in the vegetables in the same manner that it uses the form found in beef. Therefore, at this time it appears that, for vegetarians, taking supplements of vitamin B12 is an extremely good idea.

Vitamin B12 supplementation has been used with some success in treating diabetic neuropathy.[14,15] It is not clear if the success is due to the correction of a deficiency or the normalization of the deranged vitamin B12 metabolism seen in diabetics.[16] Clinically, diabetic neuropathy is very similar to that of classical cobalamin deficiency. A common symptom of cobalamin deficiency is megaloblastic anemia, anemia characterized by abnormal red blood cells in the bone marrow. Absence of megaloblastic anemia is not an adequate criteria for ruling out a deficiency of cobalamin or vitamin B12, however. A deficit within the nerve cells usually precedes anemia, often by several years. Determining the blood level of vitamin B12 is a more reliable way to diagnose a vitamin B12 deficiency than using megaloblastic anemia as an indicator.

Oral supplementation with 1,000 to 3,000 micrograms of B12 per day may be sufficient for diabetics and hypoglycemics, but intramuscular vitamin B12 may be necessary in many cases.

Vitamin E

Vitamin E functions primarily as an antioxidant. It protects against damage to the cell membranes. Without vitamin E, the cells of the body would be quite susceptible to damage. Nerve cells are particularly vulnerable. Vitamin E supplementation or a diet rich in vitamin E can protect the human body from many common health conditions, including diabetes and hypoglycemia.

Diabetics appear to have an increased requirement for vitamin E. Vitamin E not only improves insulin action, it exerts a number of beneficial effects that may aid in preventing the long-term complications of diabetes.[17] Typically, vitamin E is recommended to diabetics at a dose of 400 to 600 international units (IUs) per day. The body tolerates vitamin E extremely well, even at these high doses, but type I diabetics should start at 100 international units and raise the level 100 units per week until the desired dosage is reached. High doses of vitamin E may reduce insulin requirements.[18] Also, it is a good idea to supplement the diet with 100 to 200 micrograms of selenium whenever taking vitamin E. Selenium is a trace mineral that functions very closely with vitamin E.

Manganese

Manganese functions in many enzyme systems, including those involved in blood sugar control, energy metabolism, and thyroid function. Manganese is vital to the antioxidant enzyme superoxide dismutase, or SOD. This enzyme prevents the superoxide free radical from destroying cellular components. Without SOD, cells are quite susceptible to damage and inflammation. Manganese supplementation has been shown to increase SOD activity. Clinically, manganese is often used in the treatment of strains, sprains, and inflammation. Evidence suggests that patients with rheumatoid arthritis and, presumably, other chronic inflammatory diseases—such as diabetes—have an increased need for manganese.

Manganese is an important cofactor in the key enzymes of glucose metabolism. In guinea pigs, a deficiency of manganese results in diabetes and the frequent birth of offspring who develop pancreatic abnormalities or no pancreas at all. Diabetics have been shown to have only one-half the manganese of normal individuals. A good daily dose of manganese for a diabetic is 30 milligrams.

Magnesium

Like manganese, magnesium is involved in glucose metabolism. Considerable evidence suggests that diabetics should take supplemental magnesium. The reasons: Magnesium deficiency is common in diabetics, and magnesium may prevent some of the complications of diabetes, such as retinopathy and heart disease.[19] Of all diabetics, magnesium levels are usually lowest in those with severe retinopathy.

The RDA for magnesium is 350 milligrams per day for adult males and 300 milligrams per day for adult females. The diabetic may need twice this amount. Most of the magnesium should be derived from the diet. The average intake of magnesium by healthy adults in the United States ranges between 143 and 266 milligrams per day. This is obviously far below the RDA. Food choices are the main reason. Although magnesium occurs abundantly in whole foods, food processing "refines out" a very large portion of the element. The best dietary sources of magnesium are tofu, legumes, seeds, nuts, whole grains, and green leafy vegetables. Fish, meat, milk, and most commonly eaten fruit are quite low in magnesium. Most Americans consume a low-magnesium diet because their diet is high in refined foods, meat, and dairy products.

In addition to eating a diet rich in magnesium, the diabetic should supplement the diet with 300 to 500 milligrams of magnesium. For best results, use a highly absorbable form of magnesium, such as magnesium aspartate or citrate. Also, diabetics should take at least 50 milligrams of vitamin B6 per day. The level of vitamin B6 inside the cells of the body appears to be intricately linked to the magnesium content of the cell. In other words, without vitamin B6, magnesium will not get inside the cell and will, therefore, be useless.

Potassium

Diabetics should eat a high-potassium diet because potassium affects insulin sensitivity, responsiveness, and secretion; insulin administration induces a loss of potassium; and a high potassium intake reduces the risk of heart disease, atherosclerosis, and cancer.

Potassium is also of importance because of its role as an electrolyte. Electrolytes are mineral salts that conduct electricity when dissolved in water. Potassium is the most important dietary electrolyte. Electrolytes are required in the transmission of nerve impulses and muscle contraction. In addition to functioning as an electrolyte, potassium is essential for the conversion of blood sugar into glycogen. A potassium shortage results in a lower level of stored glycogen. Because glycogen is used by exercising muscles for energy, a potassium deficiency results in great fatigue and muscle weakness. These are typically the first signs of potassium deficiency. A potassium deficiency is also characterized by mental confusion, irritability, heart disturbances, and problems in nerve conduction and muscle contraction.

Dietary potassium deficiency is typically caused by a diet low in fresh fruits and vegetables but high in sodium. Dietary potassium deficiency is more common in the elderly than in other age groups. Dietary potassium deficiency is less common than deficiency due to excessive fluid loss (sweating, diarrhea, or urination) or the use of insulin, diuretics, laxatives, aspirin, and other drugs.

The RDA for potassium is 1.9 to 5.6 grams. If body potassium requirements are not being met through diet, supplementation is essential to good health. This is particularly true for the diabetic as well as for the elderly person and the athlete. Physicians commonly prescribe potassium salts in the range of 1.5 to 3.0 grams per day. However, potassium salts can cause nausea, vomiting, diarrhea, and ulcers. These effects are not seen when potassium levels are increased through the diet only. This highlights the advantages of using the potassium in juices, foods, or food-based supplements to meet the human body's high potassium requirements.

Most people can handle any excess of potassium. The exceptions are people with diabetes and kidney disease. These people do not handle potassium in the normal way and are more likely than others to experience heart disturbances and other consequences of potassium toxicity. Individuals with kidney disorders usually need to restrict their potassium intake and follow the dietary recommendations of their physicians. Most diabetics can consume a high-potassium diet, but they should definitely talk to their physicians about their potassium needs before taking a potassium supplement.

Zinc

Zinc is a component in over 200 enzymes in the human body. In fact, zinc functions in more enzymatic reactions than any other mineral. Although severe zinc deficiency is very rare in developed countries, many individuals in the United States have marginal zinc deficiency. This is particularly true in the elderly population. Symptoms of zinc deficiency are an increased susceptibility to infection, poor wound healing, a decreased sense of taste or smell, and skin disorders. Research suggests that zinc deficiency, like chromium deficiency, plays a role in the development of diabetes.[1]

Zinc is involved in virtually all aspects of insulin metabolism: synthesis, secretion, and utilization. Also, zinc protects against the destruction of beta-cells and has well-known antiviral effects. Diabetics typically excrete too much zinc in the urine and therefore require supplementation.[20] In experiments involving diabetic mice that took zinc supplements, all aspects of glucose tolerance improved. Zinc supplementation may have similar effects for humans. Diabetics should take at least 30 milligrams of zinc per day. In foods, zinc is found in whole grains, legumes, nuts, and seeds.

Flavonoids

The flavonoids, a group of plant pigments, are largely responsible for the colors of fruits and flowers. However, they serve more than aesthetic functions. In plants,

Table 7.2 Flavonoid Content of Selected Foods, in Milligrams, per 3½-oz (100-g) Serving

Food	4-Oxo-Flavonoids*	Anthocyanins	Catechins†	Biflavans
Fruits				
Grapefruit	50			
Grapefruit juice	20			
Oranges, Valencia	50–100			
Orange juice	20–40			
Apples	3–16	1–2	20–75	50–90
Apple juice				15
Apricots	10–18		25	
Pears	1–5		5–20	1–3
Peaches		1–12	10–20	90–120
Tomatoes	85–130			
Blueberries		130–250	10–20	
Cherries, sour		45		25
Cherries, sweet			6–7	15
Cranberries	5	60–200	20	100
Cowberries		100	25	100–150
Currants, black	20–400	130–400	15	50
Currant juice		75–100		
Grapes, red		65–140	5–30	50
Plums, yellow		2–10		
Plums, blue		10–25	200	
Raspberries, black		300–400		
Raspberries, red		30–35		
Strawberries	20–100	15–35	30–40	
Hawthorn berries			200–800	
Vegetables				
Cabbage, red		25		
Onions	100–2,000	0–25		
Parsley	1,400			
Rhubarb		200		
Miscellaneous				
Beans, dry		10–1,000		
Sage	1,000–1,500			
Tea	5–50		10–500	100–200
Wine, red	2–4	50–120	100–150	100–250

*4-oxo-flavonoids: the sum of flavanones, flavones, and flavanols.
†Catechins include proanthocyanins.
SOURCE: J. Kuhnau: The flavonoids: A class of semi-essential food components. Their role in human nutrition. World R of Nutr. and Diet 24: 117–91.

flavonoids serve as protection against environmental stress. In humans, flavonoids appear to function as "biological response modifiers."

Flavonoids seem to modify the body's reaction to compounds such as allergens, viruses, and carcinogens. In other words, flavonoids have anti-inflammatory, anti-allergic, antiviral, and anticarcinogenic properties. Recent research suggests that flavonoids may be useful in the support of many health conditions, including diabetes.[21,22] Flavonoids, such as quercetin, promote insulin secretion and are potent inhibitors of sorbitol accumulation. These actions may help explain the favorable effects of many of the botanical medicines that are used in the treatment of diabetes; these medicines are traditionally high in flavonoids. The nutritional effects of flavonoids include the ability to increase the level of vitamin C within cells, decreased leakiness and breakage of small blood vessels, prevention of easy bruising, and support for the immune system.[23] All these effects are of benefit to diabetics. In addition to consuming a diet rich in flavonoids (Table 7.2 shows the flavonoid content of certain foods), the diabetic should take an extra 1 to 2 grams of a variety of flavonoids per day.

Chapter Summary

Nutritional supplementation helps control the blood sugar level. Supplying the diabetic or hypoglycemic with additional key nutrients has been shown to improve blood sugar control as well as help prevent or improve many of the major complications of their diseases. Compared to healthy people in the general population, diabetics and hypoglycemics need more chromium, vitamin C, vitamin E, certain B vitamins, manganese, magnesium, potassium, zinc, and flavonoids.

8

Plants as Means of Blood Sugar Control

Before the advent of insulin, diabetes and hypoglycemia were treated with plant medicines. In 1980, the World Health Organization urged researchers to examine whether traditional medicines possessed any real medicinal effects. In the last 20 years scientific investigation has, in fact, confirmed the efficacy of many of these preparations, some of which are remarkably effective. The discussion in this chapter will, of necessity, be limited to a few plants—those that appear to be most effective, those that are relatively nontoxic, and those whose efficacy has been substantially documented. The following plants will be discussed: onions and garlic, bitter melon, *Gymnema sylvestre*, fenugreek, salt-bush, and pterocarpus. In addition, two other plants, bilberry and ginkgo, will be examined because of their important roles in dealing with diabetic and hypoglycemic complications.

Even though the plants discussed in this chapter can lower blood sugar, plant-based therapy should not be used by itself. Proper and effective natural treatment of diabetes and hypoglycemia requires careful integration of diet, nutritional supplements, lifestyle, and plant-based medicine. This approach is especially important in type II diabetes, which is usually the result of many years of chronic metabolic insult. Its resolution requires a comprehensive approach. The type I diabetic must carefully monitor his or her blood glucose levels during all phases of treatment, particularly if the patient has relatively uncontrolled diabetes. Careful attention to symptoms, home glucose monitoring, and the results of the glycosylated hemoglobin assay are, at this time, the best ways to monitor the progress of the diabetic individual. As the diabetic employs plant medicines as well as diet to improve blood sugar control, drug dosages will have to be altered. The patient and the prescribing doctor must work together closely.

Onions and Garlic

Onions (*Allium cepa*) and garlic (*Allium sativum*) can significantly lower the blood sugar level.[1] The active compounds in these plants are believed to be sulfur-containing compounds, allyl propyl disulfide (APDS) and diallyl disulfide oxide (allicin), although other constituents, such as flavonoids, may play a role as well.

Experimental and clinical evidence suggest that APDS lowers the glucose level by competing with insulin (also a disulfide) for insulin-inactivating sites in the liver.[2] This results in an increase of free insulin. ADPS administered in doses of 125 milligrams per kilogram to fasting humans causes a marked fall in blood glucose levels and an increase in serum insulin. Allicin, at doses of 100 milligrams per kilogram, produces a similar effect.

Graded doses of onion extract (1 milliliter of extract equals 1 gram of whole onion) at levels sometimes found in the diet (the equivalent of 1 to 7 ounces of onion), reduce blood sugar during oral and intravenous glucose tolerance tests in a dose-dependent manner. In other words, the higher the dose, the greater the effect. The effect of raw and boiled onion extracts is similar.[2]

In Chapter 10 you will read about the cardiovascular effects of eating garlic and onions—a reduction in LDL cholesterol and blood pressure. Add these benefits to the fact that eating these foods can increase serum insulin, and the message is clear: Diabetics and hypoglycemics should make liberal use of onions and garlic.

Bitter Melon

Bitter melon (*Momordica charantia*), also known as balsam pear, is a tropical fruit widely cultivated in Asia, Africa, and South America. The unripe fruit is eaten as a vegetable. Bitter melon is a green cucumber-shaped fruit, like a gourd, it has bumps all over it. It looks like an ugly cucumber. Unripe bitter melon has been used extensively in folk medicine as a remedy for diabetes.[3,4] The ability of the fresh juice or the extract of the unripe fruit to lower blood sugar has been clearly established.

Bitter melon contains several compounds with confirmed anti-diabetic properties. Charantin, extracted by alcohol, is an agent composed of mixed steroids that is more potent against hypoglycemia than the oral drug tolbutamide. Bitter melon also contains an insulinlike polypeptide, polypeptide-P, which lowers blood sugar levels when injected subcutaneously into type I diabetics.[4] Since polypeptide-P appears to have fewer side effects than insulin, it has been suggested, for some patients, as an insulin replacement. The oral administration of 2 ounces of the juice of bitter melon has produced good results in clinical trials.[3,4]

Unripe bitter melon is available primarily at Asian grocery stores. Health food stores may have bitter melon extracts, but the fresh juice is probably better to use—this was what was used in the studies. The juice of the bitter melon is, in my opinion, very difficult to make palatable. As its name implies, it is quite bitter. Simply plug your nose and take a 2-ounce shot. The dosage of other forms should approximate this dose.

Gymnema sylvestre

A plant native to the tropical forests of India, *Gymnema sylvestre* has long been used as a treatment for diabetes. Recent scientific investigation has upheld its effectiveness in treating both type I and type II diabetes.[5,6]

Gymnema sylvestre appeared on the U.S. market a few years ago. Originally it was hyped as a "sugar blocker." Manufacturers claimed that gymnema could block the absorption of sugar in the gastrointestinal tract and allow the sugar to pass through the intestines unabsorbed. Ridiculous advertisements told "how to cut down on sugar calories without cutting down on sugar." Such claims were, in my opinion, blatant distortions of truth.

Gymnema components, such as gymnemic acid, when applied to the tongue *are* able to block the *sensation* of sweetness. This has some significance. Subjects who had gymnema extracts applied to the tongue ate less at a meal, compared to those to whose tongues gymnema was not applied. Note that the people had the gymnema extract applied to their *tongues;* they did not swallow it in capsule or tablet form. Swallowing it would not necessarily produce the same effect.

In regard to diabetes, gymnema extracts have been shown to enhance glucose control in diabetic dogs and rabbits. Interestingly, in animals that have their pancreas removed, gymnema had no obvious effects. The conclusion is that gymnema enhances the production of endogenous insulin. Animal studies suggest that it accomplishes this by regenerating the insulin-producing beta cells in the pancreas. Studies of humans, both type I and type II diabetics, seem to support this.[5,6]

In one study, an extract of the leaves of *Gymnema sylvestre* was given to 27 patients with type I diabetes on insulin therapy. The effects were reduced insulin requirements, a decrease in blood sugar levels after fasting, and improved blood sugar control.[5] This study confirmed earlier work in animal studies. In type I diabetes, gymnema appears to work by enhancing the action of insulin and, as suggested, regenerating the beta cells of the pancreas.

Gymnema extract has also caused positive results in the treatment of type II diabetes.[6] In one study, 22 type II diabetics were given gymnema extract along with their oral hypoglycemic drugs. All patients demonstrated improved blood sugar control; 21 out of the 22 were able to reduce their drug dosage considerably; and 5 subjects were able to discontinue their medication and maintain blood sugar control with the gymnema extract alone.

The dosage for *Gymnema sylvestre* extract is 400 milligrams per day for both type I and type II diabetics. It is interesting to note that gymnema extract is without side effects and that it exerts its blood sugar–lowering effects only in cases of diabetes. Gymnema extract given to healthy volunteers does not produce any blood sugar-lowering or hypoglycemic effects.

Fenugreek

The seeds of fenugreek (*Trigonella foenum-graecum*) have demonstrated significant anti-diabetic effects in experimental and clinical studies.[7–9] The active ingredient is in the defatted portion of the seed and contains the alkaloid trigonelline, nicotinic acid, and coumarin.

Administration of the defatted seed (in daily doses of 1.5 to 2.0 grams per kilogram) to both normal and diabetic dogs reduced, after meals and after fasting, the levels of blood glucose, glucagon, somatostatin, and insulin, as well as total cholesterol and triglycerides. The level of HDL cholesterol increased.[7]

Human studies have confirmed these effects. Defatted fenugreek seed powder, given twice daily in a 50-gram dose to insulin-dependent diabetics, resulted in significant reduction in fasting blood sugar and improved glucose tolerance test results.[8] There was also a 54% reduction in 24-hour urinary glucose excretion and significant reductions in LDL and VLDL cholesterol and triglyceride values. In non–insulin dependent diabetics, the addition of 15 grams of powdered fenugreek seed soaked in water significantly reduced after-meal glucose levels.[9] These results indicate that the diet of the diabetic or hypoglycemic should include fenugreek seeds or defatted fenugreek seed powder.

Saltbush

Saltbush (*Atriplex halimus*), also known as sea orach, is a branchy woody shrub native to the Mediterranean area, North Africa, and Southern Europe. It is especially common around the Jordan Valley, in saline depressions and oases. Saltbush is the primary food of the sand rat. People noticed that, when sand rats switched from a diet rich in saltbush to standard rat chow, they typically developed severe diabetes. Replacing the saltbush in the diet brought about a quick reversal of the condition. Researchers began investigating the possible therapeutic benefits of saltbush for humans.

Studies conducted in Israel, which involved saltbush and human subjects, have yielded good results in patients with type II diabetes. Blood glucose levels and glucose tolerance improved. The dosage used in the human studies was 3 grams per day. Saltbush is rich in fiber, protein, and numerous trace minerals, including chromium.

Pterocarpus

Pterocarpus marsupium has a long history of use in India as a treatment for diabetes. The flavonoid epicatechin is extracted from the bark of this plant. Epicatechin has been shown to prevent beta cell damage in rats. Further, both epicatechin and a crude alcohol extract of pterocarpus have actually regenerated pancreatic beta cells in diabetic animals.[10,11] Epicatechin is also found in green tea (tea made of *Camelia sinensis*). I know of no current commercial source of pterocarpus; green tea may be a suitable alternative. Diabetics and hypoglycemics should drink at least two cups of green tea per day.

Bilberry

Bilberry (*Vaccinium myrtillus*), or European blueberry, is a shrubby perennial that grows in the woods and forest meadows of Europe. The fruit is a blue-black berry that differs from an American blueberry in that its meat is also blue-black. Bilberry-leaf tea has a long history as a folk treatment for diabetes. This use is supported by research, which has shown that oral administration reduces hyperglycemia in normal and diabetic dogs, even when glucose is injected intravenously at the same time.[12,13] Although this research is interesting, it is thought that the berries or extracts of the berries offer even greater benefit than the tea.

The active components of bilberries are flavonoids—specifically, anthocyanosides. Chapter 7 explained the importance of flavonoids in diabetes treatment. Anthocyanosides are among the most potent flavonoids. Interest in bilberry anthocyanosides was first aroused during World War II. After eating bilberries, Royal Air Force pilots reported improved night vision on bombing raids. Subsequent studies showed that the administration of bilberry extracts to healthy subjects resulted in improved nighttime visual acuity, quicker adjustment to darkness, and faster restoration of visual acuity after exposure to glare.[14]

Research also shows that anthocyanosides affect the blood vessels of the eye as well as the part of the retina responsible for vision. They can restore circulation to the retina.[14-16] Clinical studies have shown that anthocyanosides have positive results in the treatment of diabetic retinopathy, macular degeneration, cataracts, retinitis pigmentosa, and night blindness.[14,17] Bilberry extracts have been prescribed for diabetic retinopathy since 1945.

The standard dose of bilberry extract is based on its anthocyanoside content, as calculated by its anthocyanidin percentage. Widely used pharmaceutical preparations in Europe are standardized for anthocyanidin content (typically, 25%). These extracts are also available in the United States. The standard dose of an extract containing 25% anthocyanidin is 80 to 160 milligrams three times daily.

Ginkgo biloba

Medicines derived from *Ginkgo biloba* may be the most important plant-derived medicines in the world. The extract of the leaves of *Ginkgo biloba* is one of the most popular medicines in France and Germany. In Germany alone, over 5 million prescriptions for ginkgo are written each year. Unfortunately, most American physicians have never heard of it—so many Americans could benefit from ginkgo extract if their physicians knew about it. In the United States, *Ginkgo biloba* extract is available in health food stores.

The extract of *Ginkgo biloba* leaves offers great benefit to many elderly people with impaired blood flow to the brain or cerebral insufficiency.[18,19] The symptoms of cerebral insufficiency include short-term memory loss, vertigo, headache, ringing in the ears, depression, and impotence (in males). These symptoms are often referred to as "symptoms of aging." Ginkgo extract has been extensively studied and is effective in reducing all symptoms of cerebral insufficiency. Ginkgo appears to work by increasing blood flow to the brain, resulting in an increase in oxygen and glucose utilization.

Ginkgo extract has also been shown to improve the blood flow to peripheral tissues—the arms, legs, fingers, and toes. Peripheral vascular insufficiency is quite common in both diabetics and hypoglycemics. In several double-blind trials involving vascular insufficiency of the leg (intermittent claudication, see Chapter 4), ginkgo was shown to be superior to a placebo.[19-21] Not only were measurements of pain-free walking distance and maximum walking distance dramatically increased, but ultrasound measurements demonstrated increased blood flow through the affected limb.

The significance of demonstrating measurable improvement in blood flow through the affected areas is great. Although medical treatment of these patients (muscular rehabilitation and the elimination of risk factors such as smoking, excess weight, and the like) results in clinical improvement, such as increased walking tolerance, it has not shown improved perfusion of the limb, and the results are limited over time. Therefore, the muscular rehabilitation and elimination of risk factors, though valuable therapies, are not satisfactory alone.

Ginkgo is clearly an important medicine in the treatment of peripheral vascular disease due to diabetes. Ginkgo extract has also been shown to prevent diabetic retinopathy in diabetic rats, suggesting it may have a protective effect for human diabetics.[22]

To take advantage of ginkgo's effect on brain function, be sure that the product is the same as what is available in Europe. The ginkgo extract should be standardized to contain 24% ginkgo flavoglycosides (also referred to ginkgo-heterosides). The standard dosage of extract at 24% gingko flavoglycoside concentration is 40 milligrams three times per day. Ginkgo is extremely safe to use; there have been no reports of significant adverse reactions at the prescribed dosage.

Chapter Summary

Several plant-derived medicines exert effects that are of substantial benefit to people with diabetes and hypoglycemia. These herbs are effective and nontoxic. Documentation substantiates their efficacy. When a diabetic or hypoglycemic employs plant-based medicines as well as a treatment approach involving diet, nutritional supplements, and lifestyle, drug dosages will most likely have to be altered.

9

Lifestyle Factors in Blood Sugar Control

The question of health or disease often comes down to choosing a healthful alternative over a less healthful one. If you want to be healthy, simply make healthful choices. Being healthy takes commitment. The reward is often difficult to see or feel. It is usually not until your body fails you in some manner that you realize you haven't taken care of it. Many people forget that good health is a person's most valuable possession.

Diabetes or hypoglycemia is often a result of an unhealthful diet and lifestyle. The dietary aspects have been stressed throughout this book. But what about the lifestyle factors? Diet and lifestyle are intricately related. People who tend to follow a healthful diet usually have a healthful lifestyle. Conversely, people who eat a lot of sugar, also tend to smoke, drink more alcohol, and not exercise. Because of the fragile metabolic condition of diabetes, an unhealthful lifestyle is even more damaging to a diabetic than to a non-diabetic. Diabetics should avoid alcohol and cigarette smoking and incorporate exercise as part of their daily routine.

Alcohol

Alcohol consumption severely stresses blood sugar control and is often a contributing factor to hypoglycemia and diabetes. Alcohol induces reactive hypoglycemia by interfering with normal glucose utilization as well as increasing the secretion of insulin. The resultant drop in blood sugar produces a craving for food, particularly food that quickly elevates blood sugar (food containing refined sugar), as well as a craving for more alcohol. The increased sugar consumption aggravates the reactive hypoglycemia, particularly in the presence of more alcohol. Again, this aggravation is due to alcohol-induced impairment of normal glucose utilization and increased secretion of insulin.

Hypoglycemia is an important complication of acute and chronic alcohol abuse. Hypoglycemia aggravates the mental and emotional symptoms of the alcoholic and the withdrawing alcoholic. These symptoms include sweating, tremor, rapid heartbeat, anxiety, hunger, dizziness, headache, visual disturbance, decreased mental function, confusion, and depression.

Although acute alcohol ingestion induces hypoglycemia, in the long run it leads to hyperglycemia and diabetes. Eventually, the body becomes insensitive to the augmented insulin release caused by alcohol. In addition, alcohol itself can cause insulin resistance even in healthy individuals.[1] Evidence from studies of large populations indicates that alcohol intake is strongly correlated with diabetes.[2,3] The higher the alcohol intake, the more likely an individual is to have diabetes. In addition, chronic alcohol consumption is associated with heart disease, high blood pressure, some types of cancer, stroke, osteoporosis, and liver disease.

Smoking

The costs of cigarette smoking are well documented and substantial, both in terms of adverse health effects and health care expenditures.[4] (Figure 9.1 summarizes the health risks.) Yet nearly one-third of the American adult population smokes. Fortunately, the number of smokers is gradually being reduced as more and more people are becoming health conscious. It is imperative that diabetics and hypoglycemics not smoke. Diabetics and hypoglycemics are even more sensitive to the negative health effects of smoking than healthy people. Cigarette smoking greatly increases the risk of developing diabetic complications, particularly atherosclerosis. Statistical evidence reveals a three- to fivefold increase in the risk of heart disease in smokers compared to nonsmokers.[1] The more cigarettes smoked and the greater the number of years of smoking, the greater the risk of dying from a heart attack or stroke.

Cigarette smoking greatly increases the smoker's load of pro-oxidants and free radicals. Pro-oxidants, like free

---

Cardiovascular Disease
  Coronary artery disease
  Peripheral vascular disease
  Stroke

Cancer
  Lung
  Larynx, mouth, and throat
  Bladder, kidney
  Pancreas

Lung Diseases
  Cancer
  Chronic bronchitis
  Emphysema

Complications of Pregnancy
  For infants: Small size, relatively high infant mortality
  For mothers: Placenta previa, abruptio placentae

Gastrointestinal Complications
  Peptic ulcer
  Esophageal reflux

Figure 9.1   Increased risks for smokers

radicals, are highly reactive molecules that can bind to and destroy cellular components. Free radical damage is one of the major reasons we age. Also, free radical damage is linked to osteoarthritis and rheumatoid arthritis as well as the development of many other diseases. These diseases include cancer, heart disease, cataracts, Alzheimer's disease, and virtually every other chronic degenerative disease.

Although the body creates free radicals during metabolism, the environment contributes greatly to the free radical load of an individual. Many of the harmful effects of smoking are related to the extremely high levels of free radicals that are inhaled. The free radicals deplete key antioxidant nutrients such as vitamin C and beta-carotene.

Exercise

An appropriate exercise program is an important part of a diabetes or hypoglycemia treatment and prevention plan. It is well known that regular exercise can prevent type II diabetes and improve many aspects of glucose metabolism. Exercise can enhance insulin sensitivity and improve glucose tolerance in existing diabetics. Some of the effects of exercise on blood sugar control may stem from the fact that exercise increases the chromium concentration in tissue.[5]

The health benefits of regular exercise, especially for the diabetic, cannot be overstated. (Figure 9.2 summarizes the benefits.) The immediate effect is to place stress on the body. However, with a regular exercise program, the body adapts. The body's response to this regular stress is that it becomes stronger, functions more efficiently, and has greater endurance.

The entire body benefits from regular exercise largely as a result of improved cardiovascular and respiratory function. Simply stated, exercise enhances the transport of oxygen and nutrients into cells. At the same time, exercise

Improved cardiovascular function as shown by decreased heart rate, improved heart contraction, reduced blood pressure, and decreased blood cholesterol

Reduced secretions of adrenaline and noradrenaline in response to psychological stress

Improved oxygen and nutrient utilization in all tissues

Increased self-esteem, improved mood, better frame of mind

Increased endurance and energy

Figure 9.2 Health benefits of exercise

enhances the transport of carbon dioxide and waste products from the tissues of the body to the bloodstream and, ultimately, to eliminative organs.

Regular exercise is particularly important in reducing the risk of heart disease. It does this by lowering the cholesterol level, improving the blood and oxygen supply to the heart, increasing the functional capacity of the heart, reducing blood pressure, reducing obesity, and exerting a favorable effect on blood clotting.[6]

Regular exercise makes people not only look better, but also makes them feel better. Tensions, depressions, feelings of inadequacy, and worries diminish greatly with regular exercise. The value of an exercise program in the treatment of depression cannot be overstated.[7] Exercise alone has been demonstrated to have a tremendous impact on improving mood and the ability to handle stressful life situations.

How to Start an Exercise Program

The first thing to do is to make sure you are fit enough to start an exercise program. If you have been mostly inactive for a number of years or have a previously diagnosed illness, see your physician first.

If you are fit enough to begin, select an activity that gets your heart moving. Aerobic activities such as walking briskly, jogging, bicycling, cross-country skiing, swimming, aerobic dance, and racquet sports are good examples. Brisk walking (5 miles an hour) for approximately 30 minutes may be the very best form of exercise for weight loss. Walking can be done anywhere; it doesn't require any expensive equipment, just comfortable clothing and well-fitting shoes; and the risk of injury is extremely low.

Intensity of Exercise

Exercise intensity is determined by measuring your heart rate (the number of times your heart beats per minute). This can be done quickly by placing the index and middle fingers of one hand on the side of the neck just below the angle of the jaw, or on the opposite wrist. Beginning with zero, count the number of heartbeats for 6 seconds. Simply add a zero to this number and you have your pulse. For example, if you counted 14 beats, your heart rate is 140. Would this be a good number? It depends upon your training zone.

A quick and easy way to determine your maximum training heart **rate** is to simply subtract your age from 185. For example, if you are 40 years old, your maximum heart rate is 145. To determine the bottom of the training zone, simply subtract 20 from your maximum heart rate. In the case of a 40-year-old, this is 125. So, the training range for a healthy 40-year-old is from 125 to 145 heartbeats per minute. For maximum health benefits, you must stay in your training range and never exceed it.

Exercise Duration and Frequency

To gain any significant benefits from exercise, you must work for a minimum of 15 to 20 minutes, at your training heart rate, at least three times a week. It is better to exercise at the lower end of your training zone for longer periods of time than it is to exercise at a higher intensity for a shorter period of time. It is also better if you can make exercise a part of your daily routine. The key to getting the maximum benefit from exercise is to make it enjoyable. Choose an activity that you enjoy and have fun with. If you can find enjoyment in exercise, you are much more likely to exercise regularly. You don't get in good physical condition by exercising once; you must do it on a regular basis. So, make it fun.

Chapter Summary

A healthful lifestyle is critical to good health. Because diabetics and hypoglycemics are even more susceptible than others to the negative effects of alcohol consumption, cigarette smoking, and a sedentary lifestyle, it is especially important for them to choose healthful living practices.

10

Syndrome X and Cardiovascular Disease

G lucose or insulin disturbances, high blood cholesterol and triglyceride levels, elevated blood pressure, and android obesity compose a set of cardiovascular risk factors known as syndrome X. Other terms to describe this syndrome include *metabolic cardiovascular risk syndrome* (MCVS), *Reaven's syndrome, insulin resistance syndrome,* and *athero-thrombogenic syndrome.* Although there is a push to abandon the term *syndrome X,* it has nonetheless persisted.[1,2]

The underlying metabolic denominator in syndrome X is an elevated level of insulin. There is little doubt what contributes to this elevation: an elevated intake of refined carbohydrate. Early in this book, an increased refined sugar intake was said to cause hypoglycemia and later go on to cause diabetes. A recent study supports the contention that prolonged consumption of refined sugar and the resulting elevation in insulin eventually lead to type II diabetes. A 25-year research project showed that the development of type II diabetes was preceded by elevation of serum insulin and insulin insensitivity.[3] In most cases these defects presented themselves decades before the development of diabetes.

Hypoglycemia, increased insulin secretion, syndrome X, and type II diabetes can be viewed as a progression of the same illness—a malady caused by the Western diet. The human body was simply not designed to handle the amount of refined sugar, salt, saturated fat, and other harmful food compounds that many people in the United States and other Western countries feed it. The result is that a metabolic syndrome emerges—elevated insulin, obesity, elevated blood cholesterol and triglycerides, and high blood pressure. *Syndrome X* is the label that modern medicine has chosen to ascribe to a condition caused by poor dietary and lifestyle choices. It seems silly for medical researchers to be spending millions of dollars in the development of drugs ("magic bullets") instead of working on ways to aid people in choosing a more healthful diet and lifestyle.

This chapter will provide the information people with syndrome X, diabetes, or hypoglycemia need to lower blood cholesterol and blood pressure by using diet, exercise, nutritional supplements, and plant-based medicines. Foremost in the approach is the use of all the previously mentioned natural treatments for improving blood glucose control. Increased insulin and insulin insensitivity are linked to the cardiovascular complications of syndrome X and diabetes.

The Need to Lower Cholesterol

The dietary recommendations given in Chapter 6 and the lifestyle recommendations given in Chapter 9 provide the first steps toward healthful cholesterol levels. The key dietary factors are eating less saturated fat and cholesterol; increasing the consumption of fiber-rich plant foods (fruits, vegetables, grains, and legumes); and achieving ideal body weight. The lifestyle changes include getting regular aerobic exercise, stopping smoking, and reducing or eliminating the consumption of coffee (both caffeinated and decaffeinated). Since animal products are the primary sources of both saturated fats and cholesterol, it is obvious that the intake of animal products must be limited to prevent or reverse atherosclerosis. This is perhaps best illustrated in the now-famous Lifestyle Heart Trial conducted by Dr. Dean Ornish.[4] In this study, subjects with heart disease were divided into a control group and an experimental group. The control group received regular medical care while the experimental group was asked to eat a lowfat vegetarian diet for at least one year. The diet included fruits, vegetables, grains, legumes, and soybean products. Subjects were allowed to consume as many calories as they wished. No animal products were allowed except egg white and 1 cup per day of nonfat milk or yogurt. The diet contained approximately 10% fat, 15% to 20% protein, and 70% to 75% carbohydrate (predominantly, complex carbohydrate from whole grains, legumes, and vegetables).

The experimental group was also asked to perform stress-reduction techniques—breathing exercises, stretching exercises, meditation, imagery, and other relaxation exercises—for an hour each day and to exercise at least 3 hours a week. At the end of the year, the subjects in the experimental group showed significant overall regression of atherosclerosis of the coronary blood vessels. In contrast, subjects in the control group, who were being treated with regular medical care and following the standard American Heart Association diet, actually showed progression of their disease. The control group actually got worse. Ornish states "This finding suggests that conventional recommendations for patients with coronary heart disease (such as a 30% fat diet) are not sufficient to bring about regression in many patients."

Although most authorities now agree that the level of blood cholesterol is largely determined by the dietary intake of total calories of cholesterol, saturated fat, and polyunsaturated fat, the result of Ornish's study and others suggest that other factors are also important. Strict vegetarianism may not be as important as consuming a diet high in fiber and complex carbohydrates, low in fat, and low in cholesterol. It is well established, however, that vegetarians have a much lower risk of developing heart disease and a vegetarian diet has been shown to be quite effective in lowering cholesterol levels and reducing the risk for atherosclerosis.[5,6] Such a diet is rich in a number of protective factors: fiber; essential fatty acids; vitamins; and minerals, including potassium and magnesium. The dietary recommendations given in Chapter 6 are very close to the recommendations of Ornish.

Supplements That Lower Cholesterol

When there is a need for additional support to the dietary and lifestyle practices that can lower cholesterol, it simply makes sense to use natural compounds, which are actually safer and more effective than the prescription drugs commonly used for the purpose.

Niacin, or vitamin B3, has long been used to lower cholesterol. In fact, niacin is recommended by the National Cholesterol Education Program as the first "drug" to use.[7] Unlike many cholesterol-lowering drugs, which have actually been shown to reduce life expectancy, niacin can lower cholesterol safely and extend life. Niacin was the only substance to demonstrate a decreased mortality in the famed Coronary Drug Project.[8] Its effects are long-lasting, as a follow-up study to the Coronary Drug Project demonstrated. The follow-up showed that the long-term death rate for patients treated with niacin was actually 11% lower than that of the group receiving a placebo, even though the treatment for most patients had been discontinued many years earlier.[9]

Because the dose of niacin required (1 gram, 3 times per day) to lower cholesterol often results in flushing of the skin, stomach irritation, ulcers, liver damage, fatigue, and other side effects, many people are turned off by niacin. Some people combat the acute reaction of skin flushing by taking sustained-released niacin products, also called timed-released or slow-released products. These formulations allow the niacin to be absorbed gradually, thereby reducing the flushing reaction. However, though these forms of niacin reduce skin flushing, they actually have proven to be more toxic to the liver.[10]

A safer form of niacin is inositol hexaniacinate. It is composed of one molecule of inositol (an unofficial B vitamin) and six molecules of niacin. It yields slightly better results than standard niacin, but the body tolerates it much better—both in terms of flushing and, more important, long-term side effects, including effects on blood sugar control.[11-13] In fact, in one study, 153 patients were treated with inositol hexaniacinate at dosages ranging from 600 to 1,800 milligrams per day, and no patients reported any side effects or adverse reaction.[13] Based on this study and others, it appears that if people choose to self-medicate with niacin, the preferred form is inositol hexaniacinate at a dosage of 600 to 1,800 milligrams per day. Inositol hexaniacinate is available at health food stores.

Inositol hexaniacinate may offer additional benefits for people with reduced blood flow. In fact, in Europe inositol hexaniacinate is used more for its ability to improve the circulation than it is for its cholesterol-lowering effects.

Plants That Lower Cholesterol

Several plant-based medicines and plants possess impressive cholesterol-lowering qualities. The best appear to be gugulipid, garlic, and onions.

Gugulipid is the standardized extract of the mukul myrrh tree (*Commiphora mukul*), which is native to India. Several clinical studies have confirmed that gugulipid can lower both cholesterol and triglyceride levels.[14,15] Typically, with gugulipid treatment a patient's cholesterol levels will drop 14% to 27% in a 4- to 12-week period while triglyceride levels will drop from 22% to 30%.

The effect of gugulipid on cholesterol and triglyceride levels is comparable to that of lipid-lowering drugs. Those drugs are associated with some degree of toxicity; gugulipid is without side effect. Safety studies in rats, rabbits, and monkeys have demonstrated it to be nontoxic. It is also considered safe to use during pregnancy.

The dosage of gugulipid is based on its guggulsterone content. Clinical studies have demonstrated that a gugulipid extract containing up to 25 milligrams of guggulsterone per 500-milligram tablet, given three times per day, is an effective treatment for elevated cholesterol, triglycerides, or both.

Chapter 8 discussed the beneficial effects of garlic and onions for the diabetic and hypoglycemic. In addition, garlic and onions exert numerous beneficial effects on the cardiovascular system, including lowering blood lipids and blood pressure. Numerous studies have demonstrated that both garlic and onions are effective in lowering LDL cholesterol and triglycerides while raising HDL cholesterol.[16] In a 1979 population study, researchers studied three populations of vegetarians in the Jain community of India. Each population consumed differing amounts of garlic and onions. As Table 10.1 shows, the most favorable effects were observed in the group that consumed the largest amount. The study is especially significant because the subjects had nearly identical diets, except in garlic and onion ingestion.

The equivalent of 1 clove of garlic or one-half onion per day will produce good results (10% to 15% total reduction in total cholesterol levels) in most people; others may require more. Although raw is best, even cooked garlic or onion

Table 10.1   Effects of Garlic and Onion Consumption on Serum Lipids (carefully matched diets)

Garlic and Onion Consumption	Cholesterol Level	Triglyceride Level
Population 1		
Garlic 50 g/week	159 mg/dL	52 mg/dL
Onion 600 g/week		
Population 2		
Garlic 10 g/week	172 mg/dL	75 mg/dL
Onion 200 g/week		
Population 3		
No garlic or onion	208 mg/dL	109 mg/dL

produces some beneficial effects. You can also supplement your diet by using one of the wide variety of different forms of garlic that exist on the marketplace, including so-called deodorized garlic products. Use well-respected brands available at health food stores.

Summary of Guidelines for Lowering Cholesterol

The goal of therapy, whether natural or drug-based, is to get blood lipid levels down into the target range as quickly as possible. Once the target range has been achieved, begin reducing the amount of medicine by half or take it every other day. Recheck your cholesterol in one month. If the level has stabilized or continued to improve, you may no longer need the medication. If the levels have started back up again, return to the previous dosage. In all this, work closely with your physician.

The three lists that follow suggest programs to lower cholesterol naturally. Each list is specific to a particular degree of cholesterol elevation.

Mild Elevation of Cholesterol

Cholesterol: 220 to 280 milligrams per deciliter
Triglycerides: 200 to 300 milligrams per deciliter

1. Reduce excessive weight.
2. Follow the dietary guidelines in Chapter 6. Eliminate intake of cholesterol and saturated fat. Increase consumption of fiber-rich foods. Increase nut and seed consumption.
3. Exercise at least four times per week.
4. Increase garlic and onion consumption.
5. In addition to the nutritional supplements outlined in Chapter 7, supplement the diet with the following:

   Inositol hexaniacinate: 500 to 600 milligrams, three times daily.

   Flaxseed oil, 1 tablespoon daily

If, after following the preceding recommendations for three months, cholesterol has not been reduced to a satisfactory level, follow the recommendations for moderate elevation of cholesterol.

Moderate Elevation of Cholesterol

Cholesterol: 280 to 350 milligrams per deciliter
Triglycerides: 300 to 400 milligrams per deciliter

1. Employ all the measures for mild elevations of cholesterol.
2. Take one 500-milligram tablet of gugulipid extract containing up to 25 milligrams of guggulsterone, three times per day.
3. Take 5 grams of a water-soluble fiber supplement, such as psyllium seed husks or pectin, before going to bed.

Follow these guidelines for three to six months. If blood cholesterol has not dropped by at least 20%, follow the recommendations for severe elevation of cholesterol.

Severe Elevation of Cholesterol

Cholesterol: More than 350 milligrams per deciliter
Triglycerides: More than 400 milligrams per deciliter

1. Employ all the measures for moderate elevations of cholesterol.

2. Take the following nutritional supplements:
   L-carnitine: 300 to 500 milligrams, three times daily
   Pantethine: 300 to 500 milligrams, three times daily

Follow these guidelines for three months. If blood cholesterol has not dropped by at least 20%, a drug may be necessary to achieve initial control. Consult a physician. When satisfactory control over the high blood lipids has been achieved, work with the physician to taper off the medication.

The Need to Lower Blood Pressure

High blood pressure, or hypertension, refers to a blood pressure reading of greater than 140/90 millimeters of mercury. Elevated blood pressure is one of the major risk factors for a heart attack or stroke. Over 60 million Americans have high blood pressure. Approximately 38% of black adults have high blood pressure. (The rate for white adults is 29%.)

High blood pressure is closely related to lifestyle and dietary factors. Some of the important lifestyle factors that may cause high blood pressure include coffee consumption, alcohol intake, lack of exercise, stress, and smoking. Some of the dietary factors include obesity; a high sodium-to potassium-ratio; a low-fiber, high-sugar diet; a high intake of saturated fat and a low intake of essential fatty acids; and a diet low in calcium, magnesium, and vitamin C.

Besides attaining ideal body weight, perhaps the most important dietary recommendation is to increase the consumption of plant foods in the diet. Vegetarians generally have lower blood pressure levels and a lower incidence of high blood pressure and other cardiovascular diseases than nonvegetarians.[5] Although dietary levels of sodium do not differ significantly between these two groups, a vegetarian's diet typically contains more potassium, complex carbohydrates, essential fatty acids, fiber, calcium, magnesium, and vitamin C. Compared to the omnivore, the vegetarian consumes less saturated fat and refined carbohydrate.

The Role of Potassium and Sodium in High Blood Pressure

The balance between potassium and sodium is extremely important to human health. Numerous studies have demonstrated that a low-potassium, high-sodium diet plays a major role in the development of cardiovascular disease (heart disease, high blood pressure, stroke, and the like) and cancer.[17-19] Conversely, a diet high in potassium and low in sodium protects against these diseases, and in the case of high blood pressure it can be therapeutic.

Excessive consumption of dietary sodium chloride (table salt), coupled with diminished dietary potassium, is a common cause of high blood pressure. However, it is important to realize that sodium restriction alone does not improve blood pressure control in most people—sodium restriction must be accompanied by a high potassium intake.[20] In fact, in most people with high blood pressure, potassium supplementation produces better blood pressure lowering than avoidance of sodium. Nonetheless, it is the balance that is important, so sodium intake must be decreased. In American society only 5% of sodium intake comes from the natural ingredients in food. Prepared foods contribute 45% of sodium intake, 45% is added in cooking, and another 5% is added as a condiment. All that the body requires in most instances is the salt that is supplied in the food.

Most Americans have a potassium-to-sodium (K:Na) ratio of less than 1:2. This means most people ingest twice as much sodium as potassium. Researchers recommend a dietary potassium-to-sodium ratio of greater than 5:1 to maintain health. This is 10 times higher than the average intake. However, even this may not be optimal. A natural diet rich in fruits and vegetables can produce a K:Na ratio greater than 100:1, because most fruits and vegetables have a K:Na ratio of at least 50:1. For example, here are the average K:Na ratios for several common fresh fruits and vegetables:

Carrots 75:1

Potatoes 110:1

Apples 90:1

Bananas 440:1

Oranges 260:1

As mentioned in Chapter 7, potassium should be a special concern for patients with diabetes; kidney disease; and those on certain medications, including blood pressure–lowering medications. These people do not handle potassium in the normal way and are likely to experience heart disturbances and other consequences of potassium toxicity. They need to restrict their potassium intake and follow the dietary recommendations of their physicians.

Foods That Lower Blood Pressure

Foods for people with high blood pressure include celery, garlic and onions, nuts and seeds or their oils (for their essential fatty acid content), cold-water fish (salmon, mackerel, and the like), green leafy vegetables (for their calcium and magnesium), whole grains and legumes (for their fiber), and foods rich in vitamin C, such as broccoli and citrus fruits.

Celery is a particularly interesting recommendation for high blood pressure. Two researchers at the University of Chicago Medical Center have performed studies on a compound found in celery, 3-n-butyl phthalide, and found that it can lower blood pressure. In animals, a very small amount of 3-n-butyl phthalide lowered blood pressure by 12% to 14% and also lowered cholesterol by about 7%. The equivalent dose in humans can be supplied by four ribs of celery. The research was prompted by one researcher's father, who ate ¼ pound of celery every day for one week and observed that his blood pressure dropped from 158/96 to a normal reading of 118/82. The celery prescription is certainly worth a try.

Garlic and onions are also important foods for lowering blood pressure. Although most recent research has focused on the cholesterol-lowering properties of garlic and onions, both have also been shown to lower blood pressure in hypertension.[16,21] Garlic is more powerful than onion in this regard. Garlic can decrease systolic pressure by 20 to 30 millimeters of mercury and diastolic pressure by 10 to 20 millimeters of mercury. Both garlic and onions should be used liberally in the diet.

Supplements That Lower Blood Pressure

Numerous natural substances can serve as alternatives to blood pressure–lowering drugs. However, these natural alternatives are most effective when they are part of a comprehensive program that focuses on diet and lifestyle.

Population studies indicate that calcium and magnesium may offer some protection against the development of high blood pressure and heart disease.[22,23] This finding led to several clinical studies designed to determine the blood pressure–lowering effect of supplemental calcium or magnesium.[24,25] The results of these studies indicate that some people will respond to calcium or magnesium supplementation. Because this is a safe therapy, it is certainly worth a try as a step 1 medication. The dosage for calcium is 1,000 to 1,500 milligrams per day. For magnesium the dosage is 500 to 1,000 milligrams per day.

As a plant-based medication to lower blood pressure, the best appears to be hawthorn (*Crataegus oxyacantha*). Hawthorn is a spiny tree or shrub that is native to Europe. Hawthorn flowers and berries have been utilized primarily as tonics for the heart and circulatory system. The biologically active compounds are proanthocyanidins. These compounds are highly concentrated in hawthorn berry and flower extracts and are responsible for many of the health-promoting effects of hawthorn.

Hawthorn extracts are widely used by physicians in Europe and Asia to reduce blood pressure, angina attacks, and serum cholesterol levels. The mild blood pressure–lowering effects of hawthorn extracts have been demonstrated in many experimental and clinical studies.[26,27] Its action in lowering blood pressure is quite unique, in that it does so through a combination of many diverse actions. Specifically, it dilates the larger blood vessels, increases the functional capacity of the heart, and possesses mild diuretic capacity.

The dosage of hawthorn depends on the type of preparation and its source. Standardized extracts, similar to those used in Europe and Asia, are available in U.S. health food stores. These extracts are the preferred form for medicinal purposes. The dosage for a standardized hawthorn extract (which contains 1.8% vitexin-4'-rhamnoside or 10% pro-cyanidins) is 100 to 250 milligrams, three times daily. Hawthorn does not produce side effects; the body tolerates it extremely well.

The blood pressure–lowering effects of hawthorn extracts generally take two weeks to become apparent. This time is necessary for adequate tissue concentrations of the flavonoids to be achieved.

Summary of Guidelines for Lowering High Blood Pressure

Do not take high blood pressure lightly. By keeping your blood pressure in the normal range, you can not only improve the length of your life, but also the quality. This is especially true if you take natural measures, rather than drugs, to attain proper blood pressure.

The three lists that follow suggest programs to lower blood pressure naturally. Each list is specific to a particular degree of blood pressure elevation.

Mild Hypertension

140–160/90–104

1. Reduce excessive weight.
2. Eliminate salt (sodium chloride) intake.
3. Follow a healthy lifestyle. Avoid alcohol, caffeine, and smoking. Exercise and use stress-reduction techniques.
4. Follow a high-potassium diet rich in fiber and complex carbohydrates.
5. Increase dietary consumption of celery, garlic, and onions.
6. Reduce or eliminate the intake of animal fats; increase the intake of vegetable oils.

7. Supplement the diet with the following:
   Calcium: 1,000 to 1,500 milligrams per day*
   Magnesium: 500 milligrams per day*
   Vitamin C: 1 to 3 grams per day
   Zinc (picolinate): 15 to 30 milligrams per day
   Flaxseed oil: 1 tablespoon per day

*An ionized source of calcium and magnesium is most beneficial. Such sources are citrates, orotates, aspartates, or Kreb's cycle chelates.

If, after following the preceding recommendations for three to six months, blood pressure has not returned to normal, consult a physician for further nondrug recommendations.

Moderate Hypertension

140–180/105–114

1. Employ all the measures recommended for the treatment of mild hypertension.
2. Take 100 to 250 milligrams of hawthorn extract containing 1.8% vitexin-4'-rhamnoside or 10% procyanidins, three times per day.
3. Take 20 milligrams of coenzyme Q10, three times per day.

Follow these guidelines for three to six months. If blood pressure has not dropped below 140/105, work with a physician to select the most appropriate medication. If a prescription drug is necessary, calcium channel blockers or ACE inhibitors appear to be the safest.

Severe Hypertension

160+/115+

Consult a physician immediately.

Employ all the measures for mild and moderate hypertension. A drug may be necessary to achieve initial control. When satisfactory control over the high blood pressure has been achieved, work with your physician to taper off the medication.

Chapter Summary

Syndrome X is a set of cardiovascular risk factors that includes glucose or insulin disturbances, high blood cholesterol and triglyceride levels, elevated blood pressure, and android obesity. Hypoglycemia, increased insulin secretion, syndrome X, and type II diabetes can be viewed as a progression of the same illness—a malady caused by the Western diet. Most people can lower blood cholesterol and blood pressure by focusing on diet, exercise, nutritional supplements, and plant-based medicines.

11

Advice Summaries for Diabetics and Hypoglycemics

Advice for Diabetics

Proper and effective treatment of the diabetic patient requires the careful integration of a wide range of therapies. The patient for whom treatment is successful is the patient who is willing to substantially alter diet and lifestyle. Type II diabetes is usually the end result of many years of chronic metabolic insult. Although treatable with the natural metabolic approach presented here, its ultimate resolution will take persistence. Although this program is primarily designed for the type I individual, it is equally appropriate for the type II individual. The ultimate goal is to re-establish normal blood sugar control and prevent the development of diabetes or ameliorate its complications.

The diabetic, under a physician's care, must monitor himself or herself carefully, particularly if the patient is on insulin or has relatively uncontrolled diabetes. Careful attention to symptoms and the results of home glucose monitoring and other blood tests are essential. As the diabetic employs some of the suggestions described in this chapter, drug dosages will have to be altered. The patient must work closely with the prescribing physician.

Dietary Treatment for Diabetics

The high complex-carbohydrate, high-fiber diet (HCF diet), modified to incorporate more natural foods, is clearly the diet of choice in the treatment of diabetes. Avoid all simple, processed, and concentrated carbohydrates and alcohol. Eat complex-carbohydrate, high-fiber foods, and keep fats to a minimum. Legumes, onions, and garlic are particularly beneficial; consume them regularly.

Supplements for Diabetics

The following recommendations regarding the daily intake of vitamins and minerals are designed to provide an optimum intake range for maintaining the health of people with diabetes. These recommended levels are most easily attained by taking a good multiple vitamin-mineral formula and then adding specific nutrients—such as vitamin C, biotin, and niacinamide—as needed.

Vitamins for Diabetics

In the lists that follow in this chapter, you will find the abbreviation μg. This abbreviation stands for *microgram*. A microgram is one-millionth of a gram. The abbreviation IU stands for the measure known as international units.

Daily Optimal Supplementation Range for Adults

Vitamin A (retinol)	5,000–10,000 IU
Vitamin A (from beta-carotene)	10,000–75,000 IU
Vitamin D	100 IU

Vitamin E (d-alpha tocopherol)	400–1,200 IU
Vitamin K (phytonadione)	60–900 μg
Vitamin C (ascorbic acid)	2,000–9,000 mg
Vitamin B1 (thiamine)	50–100 mg
Vitamin B2 (riboflavin)	50–100 mg
Niacin	50–100 mg
Niacinamide	2,000–3,000 mg
Vitamin B6 (pyridoxine)	50–100 mg
Biotin	1–9 mg
Pantothenic acid	50–100 mg
Folic acid	400–1,000 μg
Vitamin B12	1,000–3,000 μg
Choline	150–500 mg
Inositol	250–500 mg

Minerals for Diabetics

Daily Optimal Supplementation Range for Adults

Boron	1–2 mg
Calcium	250–750 mg
Chromium	200–400 μg
Copper	1–2 mg
Iodine	50–150 μg
Iron	15–30 mg
Magnesium	350–500 mg
Manganese (citrate)	10–15 mg
Molybdenum (sodium molybdate)	10–25 μg
Potassium	200–500 mg
Selenium (selenomethionine)	100–200 μg

Silica (sodium metasilicate)	200–1,000 μg
Vanadium (sulfate)	50–100 μg
Zinc (picolinate)	15–30 mg

Plant-Based Medicines for Diabetics

Consume liberal amounts of garlic, onions, and fenugreek. If possible, drink the fresh juice of unripe bitter melon (1 to 2 ounces, three times daily), green tea or blueberry-leaf tea, and *Gymnema sylvestre* extracts. If diabetic retinopathy or peripheral vascular disease is present, take 80 to 160 milligrams of extract of bilberry (25% anthocyanidin), three times daily. Or, take 40 milligrams of extract of *Gingko biloba* (24% gingko flavoglycosides), three times per day.

Exercise for Diabetics

Develop an exercise program that reflects your interests, and implement it gradually. The program should elevate the heart rate to at least 60% of maximum for one-half hour, three times a week.

Advice for Hypoglycemics

Dietary Treatment for Hypoglycemics

The primary treatment of hypoglycemia is the use of dietary therapy to stabilize blood sugar levels. Remember, reactive hypoglycemia is not a disease, it is simply a complex set of symptoms caused by faulty carbohydrate metabolism.

All simple, processed, and concentrated carbohydrates must be avoided, while complex-carbohydrate, high-fiber foods should be stressed. Legumes should be consumed regularly. Frequent small meals may be effective in stabilizing blood sugar levels. Alcohol must be avoided as it can cause hypoglycemia.

Supplements for Hypoglycemics

The following recommendations regarding the daily intake of vitamins and minerals are designed to provide an optimum intake range for maintaining the health of those with reactive hypoglycemia. These recommended levels are most easily attained by taking a well-planned multiple vitamin-mineral formula and then adding specific nutrients—such as vitamin C and calcium—as needed.

Vitamins for Hypoglycemics

Daily Optimal Supplementation Range for Adults

Vitamin A (retinol)	5,000 IU
Vitamin A (from beta-carotene)	10,000–75,000 IU
Vitamin D	100 IU
Vitamin E (d-alpha tocopherol)	400–600 IU
Vitamin K (phytonadione)	60–900 µg
Vitamin C (ascorbic acid)	2,000–4,000 mg
Vitamin B1 (thiamine)	50–100 mg
Vitamin B2 (riboflavin)	50–100 mg
Niacin	50–100 mg
Niacinamide	50–100 mg
Vitamin B6 (pyridoxine)	25–100 mg
Biotin	100–300 µg
Pantothenic acid	25–100 mg
Folic acid	400–1,000 µg
Vitamin B12	400–1,000 µg

| Choline | 150–500 mg |
| Inositol | 150–500 mg |

Minerals for Hypoglycemics

Daily Optimal Supplementation Range for Adults

Boron	1–2 mg
Calcium	250–750 mg
Chromium	200–400 µg
Copper	1–2 mg
Iodine	50–150 µg
Iron	15–30 mg
Magnesium	250–500 mg
Manganese (citrate)	10–15 mg
Molybdenum (sodium molybdate)	10–25 µg
Potassium	200–500 mg
Selenium (selenomethionine)	100–200 µg
Silica (sodium metasilicate)	200–1,000 µg
Vanadium (sulfate)	50–100 µg
Zinc (picolinate)	15–30 mg

Plant-Based Medicines for Hypoglycemics

Refer to the section that describes plant-based medicines for diabetics, which appeared earlier in this chapter.

Exercise for Hypoglycemics

Develop an exercise program that reflects your interests, and implement it gradually. The program should elevate the heart rate to at least 60% of maximum for one-half hour, three times a week.

References

Chapter 1: Introduction to Diabetes and Hypoglycemia

Guyton AC: Textbook of Medical Physiology. Saunders, Philadelphia, 1991.

Linder MC (ed): Nutritional Biochemistry and Metabolism. Elsevier, New York, 1991.

Mahan LK and Arlin M: Krause's Food, Nutrition, and Diet Therapy, 8th edition. Saunders, Philadelphia, 1992.

National Research Council: Diet and Health. Implications for Reducing Chronic Disease Risk. National Academy Press, Washington, DC, 1989.

Wyngaarden JB, Smith LH, and Bennett JC (eds): Cecil Textbook of Medicine. Saunders, Philadelphia, 1992.

Chapter 2: Diagnosis of Diabetes and Hypoglycemia

1. Wyngaarden JB, Smith LH, and Bennett JC (eds): Cecil Textbook of Medicine. Saunders, Philadelphia, 1992.

2. Chalew SA, Koetter H, Hoffman S, et al.: Diagnosis of reactive hypoglycemia: Pitfalls in the use of the oral glucose tolerance test. Southern Medical J 79:285–7, 1986.

3. Chalew SA, McLaughlin JV, Mersey J, et al.: The use of the plasma epinephrine response in the diagnosis of idiopathic postprandial syndrome. JAMA 251:612–5, 1984.

4. Hadji-Georgopoulus A, Schmidt MI, Margolis S, et al.: Elevated hypoglycemic index and late hyperinsulinism in symptomatic postprandial hypoglycemia. J Clin Endocrinol Metabl 50:371–6, 1980.

5. Fabrykant M: The problem of functional hyperinsulinism on functional hypoglycemia attributed to nervous causes. Laboratory and clinical correlations. Metab 4:469–79, 1955.

Chapter 3: A Closer Look at Diabetes

1. Amiel SA: Intensified insulin therapy. Diabetes Metab Rev 9:3–24, 1993.

2. University Group Diabetes Program: A story of the effectiveness of hypoglycemic agents on vascular complications in patients with adult-onset diabetes. Mortality results. Diabetes 19:789–830, 1970.

3. Robertson J, Brydon WG, Tadesse K, et al.: The effect of raw carrot on serum lipids and colon function. Am J Clin Nutr 32:1889–92, 1979.

4. Yue DK, Hanwell MA, Satshell PM, et al.: The effects of aldose reductase inhibition on nerve sorbitol and myoinositol concentrations in diabetic and galactosemic rats. Metab 33:1119–22, 1984.

5. Gegersen G, Harb H, Helles A, et al.: Oral supplementation of myoinositol: Effects on peripheral nerve function in human diabetics and on the concentration in plasma, erythrocytes, urine and muscle tissue in human diabetics and normals. Acta Neurol Scand 67:164–71, 1983.

Chapter 4: A Closer Look at Hypoglycemia

1. Editorial: Statement on hypoglycemia. JAMA 223:682, 1972.

2. Cahill GF and Soelder JS: A non-editorial on non-hypoglycemia. N Engl J Med 291:905–6, 1974.

3. Reaven GM: Role of insulin resistance in human disease. Diabetes 37:1595–1607, 1988.

4. Hofeldt FD: Patients with bona fide meal-related hypoglycemia should be treated primarily with dietary restriction of refined carbohydrate. Endocrinol Metab Clin North Am 18:185–201, 1989.

5. Sanders LR, Hofeldt FD, Kirk MC, et al.: Refined carbohydrate as a contributing factor in reactive hypoglycemia. Southern Medical J 75:1072–5, 1982.

6. National Research Council: Diet and Health. Implications for Reducing Chronic Disease Risk. National Academy Press, Washington, DC, 1989.

7. Winokur A, Maislin G, Phillips JL, et al.: Insulin resistance after glucose tolerance testing in patients with major depression. Am J Psychiatry 145:325–30, 1988.

8. Wright JH, Jacisin JJ, Radin NS, et al.: Glucose metabolism in unipolar depression. Br J Psychiatry 132:386–93, 1978.

9. Schauss AG: Nutrition and behavior: Complex interdisciplinary research. Nutr Health 3:9–37, 1984.

10. Benton D: Hypoglycemia and aggression: A review. Int J Neurosci 41:163–8, 1988.

11. Virkkunen M: Reactive hypoglycemic tendency among arsonists. Acta Psychiatr Scan 69:445–52, 1984.

12. Schoenthaler SJ: Diet and crime: An empirical examination of the value of nutrition in the control and treatment of incarcerated juvenile offenders. Int J Biosocial Res 4:25–39, 1983.

13. Schoenthaler SJ: The northern California diet-behavior program: An empirical evaluation of 3,000 incarcerated juveniles in Stanislaus County Juvenile Hall. Int J Biosocial Res 5:99–106, 1983.

14. Abraham GE: Nutritional factors in the etiology of the premenstrual tension syndromes. J Repro Med 28:446–64, 1983.

15. Walsh CH and O'Sullivan DJ: Studies of glucose tolerance, insulin and growth hormone secretion during the menstrual cycle in healthy women. Irish J Med Sci 144:18–24, 1975.

16. Critchley M: Migraine. Lancet 1:123–6, 1933.

17. Dexter JD, Roberts J, and Byer JA: The five hour glucose tolerance test and effect of low sucrose diet in migraine. Headache 18:91–4, 1978.

18. Yudkin J: Metabolic changes induced by sugar in relation to coronary heart disease and diabetes. Nutr Health 5:5–8, 1987.

19. Pyorala K: Relationship of glucose tolerance and plasma insulin to the incidence of coronary heart disease: Results from two population studies in Finland. Diabetes Care 2:131–41, 1979.

20. Bansal S, Toh SH, and LaBresh KA: Chest pain as a presentation of reactive hypoglycemia. Chest 84:641–2, 1983.

21. Hanson M, Bergentz SE, Ericsson BF, et al. The oral glucose tolerance test in men under 55 years of age with intermittent claudication. Angiology June:469–73, 1987.

Chapter 5: Carbohydrates, the Glycemic Index, and Fiber

1. Koivisto VA and Yki-Jarvinen H: Fructose and insulin sensitivity in patients with type 2 diabetes. J Intern Med 233:145–53, 1993.

2. Gregersen S, Rasmussen O, Larsen S, et al.: Glycaemic and insulinaemic responses to orange and apple compared with white bread in non-insulin dependent diabetic subjects. Eur J Clin Nutr 46:301–3, 1992.

3. Rodin J: Effects of pure sugar vs. mixed starch fructose loads on food intake. Appetite 17:213–9, 1991.

4. Rodin J: Comparative effects of fructose, aspartame, glucose, and water preloads on calorie and macronutrient intake. Am J Clin Nutr 51:428–35, 1990.

5. Spitzer L and Rodin J: Effects of fructose and glucose preloads on subsequent food intake. Appetite 8:135–45, 1987.

6. National Research Council: Diet and Health. Implications for Reducing Chronic Disease Risk. National Academy Press, Washington, DC, 1989.

7. Jenkins DJA, Wolever TMS, Taylor RH, et al.: Glycemic index of foods: A physiological basis for carbohydrate exchange. Am J Clin Nutr 24:362–6, 1981.

8. Truswell AS: Glycemic index of foods. Eur J Clin Nutr 46 (supplement 2):S91–101, 1992.

9. Burkitt D and Trowell H: Western Diseases: Their Emergence and Prevention. Harvard University Press, Cambridge, MA, 1981.

Chapter 6: Dietary Guidelines and Menu Suggestions

1. Anderson J: Chapter 57: Nutrition management of diabetes mellitus. In: Modern Nutrition in Health and Disease. Goodhart R and Young VR (eds). Lea and Febiger, Philadelphia, 1988, pp. 1201–29.

2. Anderson JW and Ward K: High-carbohydrate, high-fiber diets for insulin-treated men with diabetes mellitus. Am J Clin Nutr 32:2312–21, 1979.

3. Anderson JW and Gustafson NJ: Dietary fiber in disease prevention and treatment. Compr Ther 13:43–53, 1987.

4. Simpson HCR, Simpson RW, Lousley S, et al.: A high carbohydrate leguminous fiber diet improves all aspects of diabetic control. Lancet 1:1–5, 1981.

5. Gillum RF: The association of body fat distribution with hypertension, hypertensive heart disease, coronary heart disease, diabetes and cardiovascular risk factors in men and women age 18–79 years. J Chron Dis 40:421–8, 1987.

6. Contaldo F, di Biase G, Panico S, et al.: Body fat distribution and cardiovascular risk in middle-aged people in southern Italy. Atherosclerosis 61:169–72, 1986.

7. Williams PT, Fortmann SP, Terry RB, et al.: Associations of dietary fat, regional adiposity, and blood pressure in men. JAMA 257:3251–6, 1987.

8. Haffner SM, Stern MP, Hazuda HP, et al.: Role of obesity and fat distribution in non–insulin-dependent diabetes mellitus in Mexican Americans and non-Hispanic whites. Diabetes Care 9:153–61, 1986.

9. Cheng KK, et al.: Pickled vegetables in the aetiology of oesophageal cancer in Hong Kong Chinese. Lancet 339:1314–8, 1992.

10. Cheng JT and Yang RS: Hypoglycemic effect of guava juice in mice and human subjects. Am J Chinese Med 11:74–6, 1983.

11. Singh RB, Rastogi S, Singh R, et al.: Effects of guava intake on serum total and high-density lipoprotein cholesterol levels and on systemic blood pressure. Am J Cardiol 70:1287–91, 1992.

12. Feskens EJM, Bowles CH, and Kromhout D: Carbohydrate intake and body mass index in relation to the risk of glucose intolerance in an elderly population. Am J Clin Nutr 54:136–40, 1991.

13. Mensink RP and Katan MB: Effect of dietary trans fatty acids on high-density and low-density lipoprotein cholesterol levels in health subjects. New Engl J Med 323:439–45, 1990.

14. Fraser GE, Sabaté J, Beeson WL, et al.: A possible protective effect of nut consumption on risk of coronary heart disease. Arch Intern Med 152:1416–24, 1992.

15. Sabaté J, Fraser GE, Burke K, et al.: Effect of walnuts on serum lipid levels and blood pressure in normal men. New Engl J Med 328:603–7, 1993.

16. Jostaba JN, Cruickshanks KJ, Lawler Heavner J, et al.: Early exposure to cow's milk and solid foods in infancy, genetic predisposition, and risk of IDDM. Diabetes 42:288–95, 1993.

17. Beynen AC, Van der Meer R, and West CE: Mechanism of casein-induced hypercholesterolemia: Primary and secondary features. Atherosclerosis 60:291–3, 1986.

18. Carrol KK: Review of clinical studies on cholesterol-lowering response to soy protein. J Am Dietetic Assoc 91:820–7, 1991.

19. Helgason T and Johasson MR: Evidence for a food additive as a cause of ketosis-prone diabetes. Lancet 2:716–20, 1981.

20. Schauss A: Dietary fish oil consumption and fish oil supplementation. In: A Textbook of Natural Medicine. Pizzorno JE and Murray MT (eds). Bastyr College Publications, Seattle, 1991.

21. Cobias L, Clifton PS, Abbey M, et al.: Lipid, lipoprotein, and hemostatic effects of fish versus fishoil ω-3 fatty acids in mildly hyperlipidemic males. Am J Clin Nutr 53:1210–6, 1991.

22. Stanto JL and Keast DR: Serum cholesterol, fat intake, and breakfast consumption in the United States adult population. J Am Coll Nutr 8:567–72, 1989.

23. Ripsin CM, Keenan JM, Jacobs DR, et al.: Oat products and lipid lowering, a meta-analysis. JAMA 267:3317–25, 1992.

Chapter 7: Essential Substances in Blood Sugar Control

1. Mooradian AD and Morley JE: Micronutrient status in diabetes mellitus. Am J Clin Nutr 45:877–95, 1987.

2. Anderson RA: Chromium, glucose tolerance, and diabetes. Biological Trace Element Research 32:19–24, 1992.

3. Anderson RA, Polansky MM, Bryden NA, et al.: Effects of supplemental chromium on patients with symptoms of reactive hypoglycemia. Metab 36:351–5, 1987.

4. Cunningham J: Reduced mononuclear leukocyte ascorbic acid content in adults with insulin-dependent diabetes mellitus consuming adequate dietary vitamin C. Metab 40:146–9, 1991.

5. Davie SJ, Gould BJ, and Yudkin JS: Effect of vitamin C on glycosylation of proteins. Diabetes 41:167–73, 1992.

6. Urberg M and Zemel MB: Evidence for synergism between chromium and nicotinic acid in the control of glucose tolerance in elderly humans. Metab 36:896–9, 1987.

7. Pocoit F, Reimers JI, and Andersen HU: Nicotinamide—Biological actions and therapeutic potential in diabetes prevention. Diabetologia 36:574–6, 1993.

8. Cleary JP: Vitamin B3 in the treatment of diabetes mellitus: Case reports and review of the literature. J Nutr Med 1:217–25, 1990.

9. Reddi A, DeAngelis B, Frank O, et al.: Biotin supplementation improves glucose and insulin tolerances in genetically diabetic KK mice. Life Sciences 42:1323–30, 1988.

10. Maebashi M, Makino Y, Furukawa Y, et al.: Therapeutic evaluation of the effect of biotin on hyperglycemia in patients with non-insulin dependent diabetes mellitus. J Clin Biochem Nutr 14:211–8, 1993.

11. Jones CL and Gonzalez V: Pyridoxine deficiency: A new factor in diabetic neuropathy. J Am Pod Assoc 68:646–53, 1978.

12. Solomon LR and Cohen K: Erythrocyte O_2 transport and metabolism and effects of vitamin B6 therapy in type II diabetes mellitus. Diabetes 38:881–6, 1989.

13. Coelingh-Bennick HJT and Schreurs WHP: Improvement of oral glucose tolerance in gestational diabetes. Br Med J 3:13–5, 1975.

14. Davidson S: The use of vitamin B12 in the treatment of diabetic neuropathy. J Flor Med Assoc 15:717–20, 1954.

15. Sancetta SM, Ayres PR, and Scott RW: The use of vitamin B12 in the management of the neurological manifestations of diabetes mellitus, with notes on the administration of massive doses. Ann Int Med 35:1028–48, 1951.

16. Bhatt HR, Linnell JC, and Matt DM: Can faulty vitamin B12 (cobalamin) metabolism produce diabetic retinopathy? Lancet 2:572, 1983.

17. Galli C and Socin A: Biological aspects and possible uses of vitamin E. Acta Vitaminol Enzymol 4:245–52, 1984.

18. Vogelsang A: Vitamin E in the treatment of diabetes mellitus. Ann NY Acad Sci 52:406, 1949.

19. White JR and Campbell RK: Magnesium and diabetes: A review. Ann Pharmacother 27:775–80, 1993.

20. Tarui S: Studies of zinc metabolism: Effect of the diabetic state on zinc metabolism: A clinical aspect. Endocrinol Japan 10:9–15, 1963.

21. Cody V, Middleton E, and Harborne JB: Plant Flavonoids in Biology and Medicine—Biochemical, Pharmacological, and Structure-Activity Relationships. Liss, New York, 1986.

22. Cody V, Middleton E, Harborne JB, et al.: Plant Flavonoids in Biology and Medicine II—Biochemical, Pharmacological, and Structure-Activity Relationships. Liss, New York, 1988.

23. Kuhnau J: The flavonoids: A class of semi-essential food components: Their role in human nutrition. World R Nutr and Diet 24:117–91, 1976.

Chapter 8: Plants as Means of Blood Sugar Control

1. Murray MT: The Healing Power of Herbs. Prima, Rocklin, CA, 1991.

2. Sharma KK, Gupta RK, Gupta S, et al.: Antihyperglycemic effect of onion: Effect on fasting blood sugar and induced hyperglycemia in man. Ind J Med Res 65:422–9, 1977.

3. Welihinda J, Karunanaya EH, Sheriff MHR, et al.: Effect of *Momordica charantia* on the glucose tolerance in maturity onset diabetes. J Ethnopharmacol 17:277–82, 1986.

4. Welihinda J, Arvidson G, Gylfe E, et al.: The insulin-releasing activity of the tropical plant *Momordica charantia*. Acta Biol Med Germ 41:1229–40, 1982.

5. Shanmugasundaram ERB, Rajeswari G, Baskaran K, et al.: Use of *Gymnema sylvestre* leaf extract in the control of blood glucose in insulin-dependent diabetes mellitus. J Ethnopharmacol 30:281–94, 1990.

6. Baskaran K, Ahamath BK, Shanmugasundaram KR, et al.: Antidiabetic effect of a leaf extract from *Gymnema sylvestre* in non–insulin dependent diabetes mellitus patients. J Ethnopharmacol 30:295–305, 1990.

7. Ribes G, Sauvaire Y, Baccou JC, et al.: Effects of fenugreek seeds on endocrine pancreatic secretions in dogs. Ann Nutr Metab 28:37–43, 1984.

8. Sharma RD, Raghuram TC, and Rao NS: Effect of fenugreek seeds on blood glucose and serum lipids in type I diabetes. Eur J Clin Nutr 44:301–6, 1990.

9. Mada Z, Abel R, Samish S, et al.: Glucose-lowering effect of fenugreek in non–insulin dependent diabetics. Eur J Clin Nutr 42:51–4, 1988.

10. Chakravarthy BK, Gupa S, Gambhir SS, et al.: Pancreatic beta-cell regeneration in rats by (−)–epicatechin. Lancet 2:759–60, 1981.

11. Chakravarthy BK, Gupa S, and Gode KD: Functional beta cell regeneration in the islets of pancreas in alloxan induced diabetic rats by (−)–epicatechin. Life Sciences 31:2693–7, 1982.

12. Allen FM: Blueberry leaf extract: Physiologic and clinical properties in relation to carbohydrate metabolism. JAMA 89:1577–81, 1927.

13. Bever B and Zahnd G: Plants with oral hypoglycemic action. Quart J Crude Drug Res 17:139–96, 1979.

14. Caselli L: Clinical and electroretinographic study on activity of anthocyanosides. Arch Intern Med 37:29–35, 1985.

15. Passariello N, Bisesti V, and Sgambato S: Influence of anthocyanosides on the microcirculation and lipid picture in diabetic and dyslipidic subjects. Gazz Med Ital 138:563–6, 1979.

16. Coget JM and Merlen JF: Anthocyanosides and microcirculation. J Mal Vasc 5:43–6, 1980.

17. Scharrer A and Ober M: Anthocyanosides in the treatment of retinopathies. Klin Monatsbl Augenheilkd 178:386–9, 1981.

18. Kleijnen J and Knipschild P: *Ginkgo biloba* for cerebral insufficiency. Br J Clin Pharmacol 34:352–8, 1992.

19. Funfgeld EW (ed): Rokan (*Ginkgo biloba*)—Recent Results in Pharmacology and Clinic. Springer-Verlag, New York, 1988. pp. 32–6.

20. Bauer U: Six-month double-blind randomized clinical trial of *Ginkgo biloba* extract versus placebo in two parallel groups in patients suffering from peripheral arterial insufficiency. Arzneim-Forsch 34:716–21, 1984.

21. Rudofsky VG: The effect of *Ginkgo biloba* extract in cases of arterial occlusive disease—A randomized placebo controlled double-blind cross-over study. Fortschr Med 105:397–400, 1987.

22. Doly M, Droy-Lefaix MT, Bonhomme B, et al.: Effect of *Ginkgo biloba* extract on the electrophysiology of the isolated diabetic rat retina. In: Rokan (*Ginkgo biloba*)—Recent Results in Pharmacology and Clinic. Funfgeld EW (ed). Springer-Verlag, New York, 1988. pp. 83–90.

Chapter 9: Lifestyle Factors in Blood Sugar Control

1. Hirata Y: Diabetes and alcohol. Asian Med J 31:564–9, 1988.

2. Selby JV, Newman B, King MC, et al.: Environmental and behavioral determinants of fasting plasma glucose in women. A matched co-twin analysis. Am J Epidem 125:979–88, 1987.

3. National Research Council: Diet and Health. Implications for Reducing Chronic Disease Risk. National Academy Press, Washington, DC, 1989.

4. Wyngaarden JB, Smith LH, and Bennett JC (eds): Cecil Textbook of Medicine. Saunders, Philadelphia, 1992.

5. Vallerand AL, Cuerrier JP, Shapcott D, et al.: Influence of exercise training on tissue chromium concentrations in the rat. Am J Clin Nutr 39:402–9, 1984.

6. Pollack ML, Wilmore JH, and Fox SM: Exercise in Health and Disease. Saunders, Philadelphia, 1984.

7. Farmer ME, Locke BZ, Moscicki EK, et al.: Physical activity and depressive symptomatology: The NHANES 1 epidemiologic follow-up study. Am J Epidem 1328:1340–51, 1988.

Chapter 10: Syndrome X and Cardiovascular Disease

1. Hjermann I: The metabolic cardiovascular syndrome: Syndrome X, Reaven's syndrome, insulin resistance syndrome, atherothrombogenic syndrome. J Cardiovasc Pharmacol 20(supp 8)S5–S10, 1992.

2. Maseri A: Syndrome X: Still an appropriate name. J Am Coll Cardiol 17:1471–2, 1991.

3. Martin BC, Warram JH, Krolewski AS, et al.: Role of glucose and insulin resistance in development of type 2 diabetes mellitus: Results of a 25-year follow-up study. Lancet, 340:925–9, 1992.

4. Ornish D, Brown SE, Scherwitz LW, et al.: Can lifestyle changes reverse coronary heart disease? Lancet 336:129–33, 1990.

5. Rouse IL, Beilin LJ, Mahoney DP, et al.: Vegetarian diet and blood pressure. Lancet ii:742–3, 1983.

6. Resnicow K, Barone J, Engle A, et al.: Diet and serum lipids in vegan vegetarians: A model for risk reduction. J Am Dietetic Assoc 91:447–53, 1991.

7. The Expert Panel: Report of the National Cholesterol Education Program Expert Panel on detection, evaluation, and treatment of high cholesterol in adults. Arch Intern Med 148:136–69, 1988.

8. The Coronary Drug Project Group: Clofibrate and niacin in coronary heart disease. JAMA 231:360–81, 1975.

9. Canner PL and the Coronary Drug Project Group: Mortality in Coronary Drug Project patients during a nine-year post-treatment period. J Am Coll Cardiol 8:1245–55, 1986.

10. Henkin Y, Johnson KC, and Segrest JP: Rechallenge with crystalline niacin after drug-induced hepatitis from sustained-release niacin. JAMA 264:241–3, 1990.

11. Welsh AL and Ede M: Inositol hexanicotinate for improved nicotinic acid therapy. Int Record Med 174:9–15, 1961.

12. El-Enein AMA, Hafez YS, Salem H, et al.: The role of nicotinic acid and inositol hexaniacinate as anticholesterolemic and antilipemic agents. Nutr Rep Int 28:899–911, 1983.

13. Sunderland GT, Belch JJF, Sturrock RD, et al.: A double blind randomised placebo controlled trial of hexopal in primary Raynaud's disease. Clin Rheumatol 7:46–9, 1988.

14. Satyavati GV: Gum guggul (*Commiphora mukul*)—The success story of an ancient insight leading to a modern discovery. Ind J Med Res 87:327–35, 1988.

15. Nityanand S, Srivastava JS, and Asthana OP: Clinical trials with gugulipid, a new hypolipidaemic agent. J Assoc Phys India 37:321–8, 1989.

16. Lau BH, Adetumbi MA, and Sanchez A: *Allium sativum* (garlic) and atherosclerosis: A review. Nutr Res 3:119–28, 1983.

17. Iimura O, Kijima T, Kikuchi K, et al.: Studies on the hypotensive effect of high potassium intake in patients with essential hypertension. Clin Sci 61(supp 7):77s–80s, 1981.

18. Khaw KT and Barrett-Connor: Dietary potassium and blood pressure in a population. Am J Clin Nutr, 39:963–8, 1984.

19. Skrabal F, Aubock J, and Hortnagl H: Low sodium/high potassium diet for prevention of hypertension: Probable mechanisms of action. Lancet ii:895–900, 1981.

20. Meneely G and Battarbee H: High sodium–low potassium environment and hypertension. Am J Cardiol 38:768–81, 1976.

21. Foushee D, Ruffin J, and Banerjee U: Garlic as a natural agent for the treatment of hypertension: A preliminary report. Cytobios 34:145–52, 1982.

22. McCarron DA and Morris CD: Epidemiological evidence associating dietary calcium and calcium metabolism with blood pressure. Am J Nephrol 6(supp 1):3–9, 1986.

23. Whelton PK and Klag: Magnesium and blood pressure: Review of the epidemiologic and clinical trial experience. Am J Cardiol 63:26G–30G, 1989.

24. Sowers JR, Zemel MB, Standley PR, et al.: Calcium and hypertension. J Lab Clin Med 114:338–48, 1989.

25. Motoyama T, Sano H, and Fukuzaki H: Oral magnesium supplementation in patients with essential hypertension. Hypertension 13:227–32, 1989.

26. Ammon HPT and Handel M: Crataegus, toxicology and pharmacology. Planta Medica 43:101–20, 318–22, 1981.

27. Murray MT: The Healing Power of Herbs. Prima, Rocklin, CA, 1991.

Index

Menopause is a natural part of life, and the way you deal with it should be too. Dr. Michael Murray, one of the world's foremost authorities in nutritional and natural medicine, presents a natural approach to deal with the effects of menopause. He covers topics such as:

- the causes of menopause
- the benefits and risks of estrogen replacement therapy
- herbal remedies and natural foods that can control symptoms
- vitamins and minerals to enhance circulation

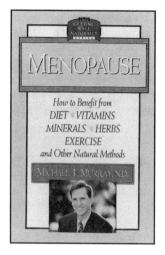

Your sexual vitality is important to you and to the one you love. It encompasses both performance and fertility and affects the way you feel about yourself. In *Male Sexual Vitality*, Dr. Michael Murray suggests a natural approach to regaining and maintaining your energy. He covers topics such as:

- specific nutrients for optimal sexual function
- understanding impotence
- causes and treatments for low sperm count
- natural herbs for enhanced libido and performance— regardless of age

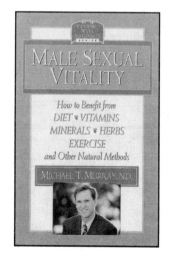

FILL IN AND MAIL TODAY

PRIMA PUBLISHING
P.O. BOX 1260BK
ROCKLIN, CA 95677

USE YOUR VISA/MC AND ORDER BY PHONE:
(916) 632-4400 (M-F 9:00-4:00 PST)

Please send me the following titles:

Quantity	Title	Amount
_____	*Menopause* $12.95	_____
_____	*Male Sexual Vitality* $11.00	_____
_____	_____	_____
_____	_____	_____
_____	_____	_____

Subtotal $_____

Postage & Handling
($4.00 for the first book
plus $1.00 each additional book) $ _____

Sales Tax
7.25% Sales Tax (California only)
8.25% Sales Tax (Tennessee only)
5.00% Sales Tax (Maryland only)
7.00% General Service Tax (Canada) $_____
TOTAL *(U.S. funds only)* $_____

❏ Check enclosed for $_____(payable to Prima Publishing)

      Charge my   ❏ Master Card   ❏ Visa

Account No. _____Exp. Date _____

Signature _____

Your Name _____

Address _____

City/State/Zip _____

Daytime Telephone _____

Satisfaction is guaranteed— or your money back!
Please allow three to four weeks for delivery.
THANK YOU FOR YOUR ORDER